OXFORD MEDICAL PUBLICATIONS

Talking with Patients

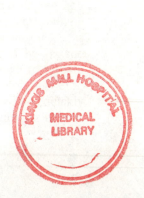

Talking with Patients
Keys to Good Communication

THIRD EDITION

PHILIP R. MYERSCOUGH
FRCS Ed, FRCP Ed, FRCOG
*Hon. Fellow, Department of Obstetrics and Gynaecology,
University of Edinburgh*

and

MICHAEL J. FORD
MD, FRCP Ed
*Consultant Physician, Eastern General Hospital,
Hon. Senior Lecturer, Department of Medicine,
University of Edinburgh*

With Contributions by

C.T. CURRIE
Senior Lecturer in Geriatric Medicine, University of Edinburgh

D. DOYLE
Medical Director, St Columba's Hospital, Edinburgh

A.N.M. HEWITT
General Practitioner and Associate Adviser in General Practice

I.A. LAING
*Senior Lecturer (P/T), Department of Child Life and Health,
University of Edinburgh*

A.L. SPEIRS
*former Consultant Paediatrician, Royal Hospital
for Sick Children, Glasgow*

R.M. WRATE
Consultant in Adolescent Psychiatry, University of Edinburgh

OXFORD
UNIVERSITY PRESS

OXFORD

UNIVERSITY PRESS

Great Clarendon Street, Oxford OX2 6DP

Oxford University Press is a department of the University of Oxford.
It furthers the University's objective of excellence in research, scholarship,
and education by publishing worldwide in

Oxford New York

Athens Auckland Bangkok Bogotá Beunos Aires Calcutta
Cape Town Chennai Dar es Salaam Delhi Florence Hong Kong Istanbul
Karachi Kuala Lumpur Madrid Melbourne Mexico City Mumbai
Nairobi Paris São Paulo Singapore Taipei Tokyo Toronto Warsaw

with associated companies in Berlin Ibadan

Oxford is a registered trade mark of Oxford University Press
in the UK and in certain other countries

Published in the United States
by Oxford University Press Inc., New York

First edition published 1989
Second edition published 1992
Third edition published 1996
Reprinted 1999, 2001

A catalogue record for this book is available from the British Library

Library of Congress Cataloging in Publication
(Data available)

ISBN 0 19 262570 5

Printed in Great Britain
on acid-free paper by
Biddles Ltd, *www.biddles.co.uk*

Preface to the Third Edition

This new edition maintains the author's original aim of helping those embarking on clinical work to develop their communication skills. The need for education and training in this field is now recognized in British medical schools, but the courses which are evolving to meet this objective have to compete for time and resources within the core of an already crowded curriculum. Few medical teachers have themselves been formally trained to teach communication skills—most are self-taught enthusiasts—and their students are likely to encounter in the rest of their training, a great diversity of role models, not all of them beneficial.

At the same time, in the public perception, the notions of individual autonomy and of 'patients' rights' exert growing influence, and patients' expectations continue to rise. Doctors' communication skills are exposed to constant scrutiny, and have attracted measured public criticisms from the National Health Service Commissioner (Ombudsman) and the Audit Commission, referred to elsewhere in the text.

The efforts to improve the teaching of doctor–patient communication have gained ground during a period of major organizational change in the National Health Service. In hospitals, more rapid turnover has been accompanied by shorter periods of duty for junior doctors, and now by the prospect of shorter but more intensive specialty training. The time available to learn and practise sensitive communication is under pressure, and the spread of high-technology care creates a more hectic and impersonal environment, in which monitors and other instruments provide a great deal of vital immediate information about patients, which appears to bypass and overshadow the need for much interpersonal dialogue. To quote from a leading article in the British Medical Journal on the importance of clinical skills [127] 'We must heed the desperate voice of the patient trapped in technology, crying 'Speak to me!''.

However, these pressures within the learning environment also highlight the importance of good communication if errors and misunderstandings are to be avoided. As the complexity and potential of modern therapy grows, the provision of adequate information for patients and their relatives, and the responsibility for securing informed consent alike become issues of greater concern.

Besides, a Report of a joint working party of the Royal Colleges of Physicians and Psychiatrists [128] has emphasized that up to half of all new hospital outpatients are suffering from psychological problems which may trigger physical symptoms without disease being present. 'Lack of privacy, lack of time, and the fact that modern medicine is overwhelmingly geared towards physical illness often result in these problems being inadequately recognized and treated.'

I am delighted to be joined by Dr Mike Ford, a general physician of wide experience, as co-author. He has contributed new sections covering some of those areas which provide a challenge to communication skills. I also welcome the help of two other new contributors. Dr Ninian Hewitt has written the chapter on communication in primary care, and Dr Iain Laing has written on talking about babies.

The text has undergone general revision, and certain sections have been expanded, notably those on body language, breaking bad news, palliative care, disability, pain, and patient information. New references have been included. I have continued to use the term 'him' in most instances when referring to the doctor or the patient. Although I recognize that some may feel this is insensitive, I have not succeeded in finding a simple alternative form of words.

As well as acknowledging the contributions of my colleagues, I also wish to express my indebtedness to those others among whose thoughts and writings I have gleaned, in an attempt to provide a broader approach than can be derived from personal experience alone. I also wish to thank the reviewers of the earlier edition, whose criticisms and suggestions have been very helpful.

I am grateful, too, for the friendship of colleagues in many countries, through whom I have caught glimpses of their cultures; and to a former patient, Mrs Isobel Paris, who has provided living lessons not only in coping with severe choreo-athetoid spastic diplegia, but also in coping with attitudes to disability.

Edinburgh   P.R.M.
July 1995   M.J.F.

Preface to the First Edition

This book has been written primarily for medical students who are embarking on clinical work. It will also be helpful reading for senior students and young doctors who are aiming to improve their communication skills and so to prepare a sound foundation for a career in any branch of clinical medicine. The author and his contributors have endeavoured to set out in a clear and concise manner the elements that promote good communication, and the skills through which these are deployed in day-to-day practice.

This area of learning is of equal importance for students of nursing, and of other health professions, particularly those whose work involves touching as well as talking. It is not assumed that the reader already has any great depth of knowledge of either clinical or behavioural science. Although the focus of the volume is on the verbal interaction between patient and doctor—the medical interview—the skills described can readily be applied in other professional settings.

As well as interpersonal dialogue, other dimensions of communication are discussed, including written communication. A recurring theme throughout the book is the manner in which the doctor (or other health professional) can facilitate or, regrettably, inhibit the expression by the patient of the feelings and concerns that are likely to arise during illness.

The need for medical training to include greater emphasis on communication skills is now becoming widely recognized. The Education Committee of the General Medical Council underlined this need in its Recommendations (1980), and made communication the topic of its annual educational symposium in 1987. The Royal College of Physicians of London has given notice that assessment of communication skills will in future from part of the Membership examination. The Royal College of Physicians of Edinburgh has recently promoted a major symposium on this topic. From the other side of the fence, the Patients Association and other groups representing clients regularly express their concern that doctors and other health professionals should learn to communicate better.

In most of the text both the patient and the doctor are referred to as 'he' rather than the more cumbersome 'he or she' in every instance. This in no way implies any intention of devaluing the female sex, or ignoring the role of women in medicine. It is merely a convenience of style.

I am greatly indebted to the four colleagues who have each contributed a chapter in their own areas of special expertise. This has brought to the book a breadth and diversity that it would not otherwise have achieved. They are:

Dr A.L. Speirs, *OBE, MD, FRCP (London and Glasgow), DCH, former Consultant Paediatrician, Royal Hospital for Sick Children, Glasgow, Stirling Royal Infirmary, and Falkirk and District Royal Infirmary.*

Dr R.M. Wrate, *DPM, FRC Psych, Consultant in Adolescent Psychiatry. Hon. Senior Lecturer, Department of Psychiatry, University of Edinburgh.*

Dr C.T. Currie, *FRCP Ed, Senior Lecturer in Geriatric Medicine, University of Edinburgh.*

Dr D. Doyle, *OBE, FRCS Ed, FRCP Ed, FRCGP, Medical Director, St Columba's Hospice, Edinburgh.*

My thanks are also due to my former departmental colleague Dr Tony Bramley, who provided the line drawings.

Oman P.R.M.
June 1988

Contents

1 Introduction

Most medical students approach their training with a desire to help people. Thus, from the very beginning of their studies, students look forward to clinical involvement—to meeting 'real' patients and learning to interact with them. After qualifying, most doctors spend a great deal of their working time communicating with patients—speaking, listening, responding. This face-to-face interaction, with exchange of information, is essential if the doctor is to be effective in his or her work.

Accordingly, skilful communication has become widely recognized as a primary component of medical education, something that the student should learn about as a basic part of professional training. However, this is the very aspect of doctors' professional skills that is still the most common cause of complaint from patients or their relatives, an apparent weak point in doctors' professional competence [1,9,10,11,12,13].

Patients single out the affective dimensions of communication in particular as unsatisfactory: some doctors are regarded as people with whom it is difficult to talk about the feelings associated with illness. Conversely, patients' feelings of satisfaction after consultations often relate to the doctor's friendliness, his understanding of their expectations, and his ability to handle their worries and concerns [2,3,4].

Only recently have considered attempts been made to teach communication skills to medical students in Britain. Traditionally, doctors have developed such facility for communication as they possess by trial and error as they practised. The need to acquire the relevant professional knowledge, skills and attitudes—to learn the scientific basis from which the art of competent communication is derived—has gradually been recognized.

Initially, the efforts tended to be scattered within the curriculum, fairly limited in scope, and did not include formal assessment. By

1993, however, a survey for the *Student British Medical Journal* found that only one British medical school did not provide a specific course in communication skills. The current pattern of such training commonly comprises a short one-off course (averaging 20 hours in total) led by psychiatrists, behavioural scientists, and/or general practitioners, since it has been in these departments that the importance of these skills was first recognized, and teaching experience developed. But the survey noted that only two schools had staff who had been trained for such teaching, despite the fact that many of them found it a 'difficult area'. However well conducted these courses are, students may regrettably come to believe that the skills concerned are relevant only or mainly in the particular circumstances of psychiatric or general practice.

In this book, therefore, I have attempted to underline the relevance of communication skills in all areas of medicine. At the same time, I have tried to distil the essential elements into a concise form, as free as possible from the jargon of the behavioural sciences and the mystique of educational theory, to aid the student who seeks to develop skill as a communicator. While it is intended primarily to be of assistance to undergraduates, I hope it will interest practising doctors who are alive to the need for continued learning.

BENEFITS FROM COMMUNICATION SKILLS

Before going further, it is worthwhile to look at the benefits that can accrue from developing interviewing skills. Good communication is not an esoteric theoretical objective, nor is it just about becoming a more understanding and approachable doctor (though that is a likely bonus). It is about being a more efficient doctor. Communication is, to put it simply, the key to effectiveness for the doctor as a professional.

First, communication skill is an absolute requirement in obtaining from the patient an authentic account of his illness as he has experienced it (the history). This information alone, if gathered and assessed with care, provides a correct diagnosis in more than a half of all patients [5], and in as many as four out of five general medical cases [6]. Without good communication, errors of diagnosis and unnecessary investigations are more likely.

Second, communication skill constitutes one of the cornerstones of therapy. Most consultations end with some sort of conclusion from the doctor, that may be called the *exposition* [7], during which the doctor offers his assessment of the case and outlines proposed treatment. As well as a clear grasp of the doctor's instructions, rapport, confidence, and trust are necessary for the patient to respond to the doctor's advice, understand the nature of his illness, comply with specific recommendations made, take (and continue to take) any medication prescribed, and be willing to return if he continues to have problems. These elements in the relationship also have therapeutic value, and may contribute directly to the patient's recovery. Without them, poor compliance is more likely.

Commonly, too, a doctor's recommendations include educational advice aimed at modifying the patient's way of life—advice to change eating patterns, take more exercise or rest, avoid recourse to alcohol, curtail smoking, avoid certain forms of stress, and so on. This educational advice and counselling can be expected to have an impact only if the relationship between doctor and patient rests on mutual confidence and respect, and if the patient's attitude to his illness is known and understood by the doctor.

Good communication between doctor and patient indirectly affords a further important benefit, for the doctor at least: it makes it much less likely that dissatisfaction with the doctor's professional services will end in litigation. The experience of the medical protection societies has provided clear evidence that, although no doctor is immune from making a mistake, a lawsuit is much more likely when communication between doctor and patient, or between doctor and doctor, has been poor. Their experience also underlines the protective value of good written communication in the patient's records and in correspondence between doctors. The important function of the written record is discussed later.

In many areas of contemporary practice, the best results are obtained only by the co-operative efforts of a co-ordinated team with different disciplinary skills. It is worth emphasizing, as Enelow and Swisher have done [8], that doctors can only exercise leadership within a group of caring professionals through their ability to function as the principal communicators. Unless that role is competently performed, any claim to leadership is a sham.

POOR COMMUNICATION

So much for the positive side of the coin. When the effects of poor communication are considered, it becomes even more clear that communication is at the heart of a sound doctor–patient relationship. As already indicated, when patients have the opportunity to criticize their doctors, their dissatisfactions usually centre not around the doctor's technical competence, but around his inadequacies as a communicator. The sorts of criticism that are expressed have been summarized in numerous published reports, including those of Cartwright [9], Dunkelmans [10], Hawkins [11], Parkin [12], and Reynolds [13]. They are concerned with doctors' unapproachability and with the inadequate explanations that patients often feel they are given regarding investigations undertaken when they are unwell and the nature of their illnesses [11,14].

'My doctor? Oh, he's thorough enough, but he's not the listening sort. I couldn't talk to *him* about *that!*'

'Of course, they looked after me superbly in hospital, but they never actually *tell* you *anything*. And you don't like to ask, do you?'

'He just gave me the prescription, and out I came. Nothing was said about what's *really* wrong with me. And I never got a chance to try and tell him how I was feeling.'

The 1991 Report of the NHS ombudsman [15] stressed that 90 per cent of the cases dealt with stemmed from failures of communication rather than poor medicine. Not only were doctors among the worst communicators, but slapdash medical record keeping, with undated, untimed, and illegible entries, or no entries at all relating to significant events during hospital stay were also criticized.

In contemporary practice, more and more patients want to be involved in decisions about their own bodies, and to participate intelligently in their own care and treatment. This is an inevitable and wholly desirable consequence of improved education and greater health consciousness among the population. It is demonstrated by the popularity of organic and health foods, health clubs, health magazines, and activities such as jogging and aerobics, not to mention the proliferation of alternative forms of medicine.

The deficiencies, then, identified by some patients relate particularly to the handling of the affective aspects of health and illness, to discussion of their close personal relationships, or of their emotional reactions to ill health: anxiety about disability, pain, loss of employment, or death, are some of the more serious concerns.

OBSTACLES TO COMMUNICATION

Among the topics which are difficult to talk about, two are associated with particular reticence. Death and sexuality are identified as 'problem' topics that are difficult to discuss with patients by both medical students [16] and junior doctors [17]. These are subjects which most human beings find it difficult to speak about openly and honestly, even with close friends. This aversion is greatly intensified when the prospect of death or sexual dysfunction has become a personal threat to the patient's well-being.

There are, of course, very many medical interviews in which neither death and suffering nor sexuality enter the dialogue in any way whatsoever. But the inhibitions that surround these topics specifically are such that they can lead to a general reluctance to become involved with *any* of the patient's feelings or personal relationships. In consequence, a greater distance is maintained in the professional relationship.

Besides, there are particular reasons why doctors find difficulty in talking about death and sexuality in a professional context. Later chapters review in more detail the reasons why these topics are such sensitive areas, and consider ways in which such sources of 'discomfort' can be handled with greater ease and skill.

It can be argued that the apparent disparity between some doctors' technical competence on the one hand, and their skill in handling the affective aspects of illness on the other, is simply a reflection of the traditional dominance of the physical sciences in pre-clinical teaching, largely at the expense of applied behavioural science. The imbalance, a legacy perhaps of the educational 'model' advocated by Flexner [18], is slowly changing, but this is not the whole story. It will become evident that a number of other important factors can make the doctor ill at ease with patients' feelings, and therefore reluctant to discuss or take account of them.

Doctors' avoidance of emotive or painful topics can be an unconscious defence against a cumulative burden of stress, which in some measure they cannot evade. It is associated with higher levels of suicide, alcoholism, drug addiction, and marital breakdown among doctors than in any other occupational group. Ways in which doctors can protect their own well-being are discussed in later chapters.

2 Doctors' and patients' roles

To understand more clearly how doctors and patients interact, it is helpful to specify what is special about the doctor–patient relationship. Just as the pattern of communication affects a relationship, so the relationship, in a circular interaction, shapes and influences the manner of communication. How do the doctor and the patient, as they interact, view themselves and one another?

Pendleton *et al.* [19] describe and discuss six ways of studying the interaction between doctor and patient. These are (1) medical; (2) sociological; (3) anthropological; (4) transactional; (5) social psychological; (6) psychoanalytical. The different behavioural sciences direct attention to particular features of the roles and behaviours of the doctor and the patient. Interviews may be studied by categorization of utterances and phrases; by finely focused discourse analysis; by psychoanalytic interpretations, or by study of non-verbal behaviour. Given this diversity of viewpoints, a panoramic catholic approach seems appropriate here, to provide a broad basis of understanding. Let us consider the patient first.

THE SICK ROLE

By speaking of the patient's role as that of a sick person, the intention is not to present a stereotyped view of how a patient does or should react to illness. On the contrary, the reader is likely to have recognized already that different individuals react in very different ways when they feel, or think they are, ill.

However, most people who are unwell look to the doctor for help, advice, or reassurance, and so they assume, as a sick person, a dependent role. This 'submission' to their medical attendant derives from the feelings of uncertainty and fear that come with illness. In turn, the patient's dependence tends to boost the doctor's self-assurance. Such words as 'I am in your hands, doctor. I'll just take your advice' do a great deal for the doctor's morale.

Occasionally, the patient is so anxious to be helpful to the doctor (and thereby to speed recovery) that he may be reluctant to deny having *any* symptom that is mentioned to him during questioning, and thus may seriously mislead the doctor. For this reason, 'leading' questions that invite a particular answer should be avoided, especially when the patient is initially describing his complaints.

Sometimes, patients are only too ready to adopt the sick role as a means of escape from the pressures of life, at home or at work. Others find being 'unwell' the only sure way of gaining the attention and concern of those around them; these attention-seekers may enjoy recurrent ill health for year after year! Children, too, may feign or exaggerate illness as an escape from school.

The close attention which those who are very ill may receive itself readily induces dependency. Patients recovering after intensive care commonly experience a reaction to withdrawal of care, and may feel for a time neglected—and resentful.

The dependency and submissiveness shown by many patients carries with it a danger of promoting a paternalistic attitude, which the doctor must guard against, since it may lead him to overlook the patient's wishes and concerns, as he pursues his own professional agenda.

Among the more strange historical examples of sickness behaviour is the story of Florence Nightingale, who, after displaying immense courage, determination, and capability during her nursing career, took to her bed and remained there for a considerable part of her life, although still in good physical health. Another bizarre pattern is seen in the so-called Münchausen syndrome [20]. Occasionally, individuals are encountered in various fields of practice who repeatedly, and often very cunningly, secure admission to hospital by falsifying the signs and symptoms of serious disease in themselves or, even more strangely, in their children [21].

In contrast, a few patients find difficulty in acknowledging that they are ill, and resist the sick role. Some of them are playing the ostrich, and refusing to face the possibility of disability or death. Some are acting bravely to try to protect their spouse or other loved ones from being upset by possible bad news. It is noteworthy that those whose everyday work centres on physical fitness, such as physiotherapists, athletes, physical instructors, and professional soldiers, as well as 'fitness freaks', often find the greatest difficulty in coming to terms with the idea that they are unwell. They regard health with such positive value that they are reluctant to acknowledge the fact of being ill.

THE DOCTOR'S 'PROFESSIONAL' ROLE

Doctors are likely to believe that the essential practical core of their professional role is (1) to diagnose—to find out what is wrong—to assign a medical label; and (2) to treat—to prescribe, advise, or perform treatment. These objectives comprise the doctor's agenda in most consultations.

The notion of being a professional has several different dimensions. It signifies an area of competence, within which the professional has both responsibility and limited authority, and so a doctor is expected to take charge of the interview with his patient and to be capable of helping him. It also signifies a degree of controlled concern for the client (patient) but at the same time a formality, an unemotional correctness of manner, and a degree of detachment. To call a relationship 'professional' is to imply that it lacks the open feeling and warmth of a normal human relationship. Hence, the SAS man, after taking out a few terrorists in an eruption of ruthless violence, is spoken of as 'doing a professional job'.

Now if the term 'professional' can convey these overtones of detachment, the word 'clinical' has also, in general parlance, come to imply even more strongly a cool, almost indifferent competence. Thus, when a few years ago a prisoner was executed in Florida in the electric chair in the presence of public representatives, their leader was happy to emerge afterwards and reassure waiting reporters that it had all been carried out 'clinically'! Similarly, an RAF Squadron Leader, during debriefing after a low-level bombing sortie, said, 'You feel very clinical—terribly clinical . . . I would not be doing this job if I was worried about it. You have got to control your emotions'. These episodes illustrate vividly the ordinary person's appreciation of the clinical atmosphere that doctors can unwittingly create—efficient certainly, but aloof, depersonalized, and unfeeling.

Why, then, do these insensitive attributes come to be associated with doctors' day-to-day working style, so providing some grounds for the criticisms, referred to in Chapter 1, that patients sometimes make of medical practitioners? It could be argued that, even from the patients' point of view, a degree of controlled clinical detachment is necessary to create the freedom for patients to share their problems with a doctor, knowing therefore that he is not being expected to shoulder the whole burden of their distress.

It is essential to understand more clearly the nature of the balance between detachment and involvement if doctors are to become better communicators, and if the divergence between patients' needs and expectations and doctors' apparent performance is to be reconciled. To do this, it is helpful to look at the factors that significantly influence doctors' professional behaviour, and that therefore shape their clinical style and determine their ability to become involved with the affective aspects of illness.

FACTORS INHIBITING COMMUNICATION

There are several factors that, consciously or unconsciously, may inhibit affective communication between doctor and patient. The first and simplest is *time*, or the lack of it. For most doctors, time is a precious commodity which has to be rationed out over the commitments of the day, while some is kept in reserve for the unexpected 'extra'. This pressure of time inevitably creates a reluctance on the part of the doctor to become involved in peripheral matters, inessentials, or irrelevancies. The patient's personal concerns may (unfortunately) be seen as falling into these categories.

Patients are likely to be inhibited from expressing their worries and other feelings by the sense that the doctor is short of time. If there are other patients sitting in the waiting room, it may seem selfish to take up what they feel is a disproportionate share of the doctor's time. So they may feel guilty and reluctant to talk.

'You're always such a busy person, doctor. I don't want to take up more of your time today.'

'I'm sure you've got more important things to attend to than my little worries.'

As well as this practical problem of pressure of time, two other factors already mentioned, can inhibit affective communication between doctor and patient because of the uncomfortable, and at times intolerable, feelings that they are able to endanger within the professional relationship. These are suffering and death on the one hand, and sexuality on the other.

Death and suffering

All doctors need some protective insulation from the distressing feelings that pain, suffering, and death inevitably evoke during the course of serious illness. These emotions are especially difficult for doctors to live with because they are likely to feel that it is their professional responsibility to prevent suffering, and that death in particular is the ultimate failure in medical practice.

But whatever the doctor's attitudes towards death and suffering, he cannot be expected to carry the burden of the distress created by illness, and may find he can protect himself from these painful feelings by avoiding involvement in any of the affective aspects of his patients' ill health. In consequence, he has distanced himself from the patient as a person, so that he can feel less closely involved. Maguire [22] described how both doctors and nurses usually distance themselves from patients who are terminally ill, to ensure their own emotional survival.

Sexuality

A second source of professionally unacceptable or intolerable feelings is sexuality. Clinical practice regularly exposes doctors to degrees of nudity and intimate forms of touching that in any other private setting would be permitted only to a lover and could be associated with sexual arousal (Fig. 2.1). This intimacy of clinical practice has to be professionalized to render it secure and emotionally comfortable for both doctor and patient. How this is achieved is not taught explicitly, but is usually learnt by example. A great deal of the impersonal formality of doctors' professional style relates to the need to desexualize the closeness of clinical contact (see p. 51).

In various ways, then, doctors contrive to become indifferent to nudity and intimate touching in a professional setting. However, they may achieve this professionalism only through an unwillingness to think about the patient as a sexual person, thereby

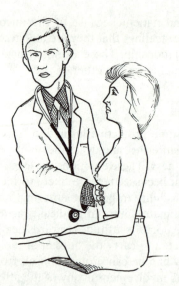

Fig. 2.1 Coping with the intimacy of clinical examination. Note the avoidance of eye contact

excluding the patient's sexuality from consideration or discussion. At the worst, these influences can mean that the doctor eliminates all warmth from his professional manner, and in some instances make open discussion of sexual problems unthinkable for him.

Because an understanding of the part these factors play in inhibiting effective communication is important, I shall return to them at a later stage.

THE WARD ENVIRONMENT

Those who are starting to work in hospital may not at first recognize that the ward environment itself should be included among the potential obstacles to good communication between patient and doctor. When patients are admitted to a ward, they sense that they have, willy-nilly, become part of a close-knit group. They quickly begin to recognize the daily routines of life in the ward, to which they are expected to conform. They cannot fail to become aware of other patients, some of whom may be more ill than themselves. At the same time, they can readily see how busy the medical and nursing staff are as they cope with the pace of more rapid turnover.

In such an environment, patients almost inevitably feel under pressure not to be too demanding, not to take up too much of the staff's time, to contain their worries, and certainly to express them only to the 'correct' person at the proper time. Both patients and staff tend to have an image of the 'good' patient—helpful, pleasant, and, as far as possible, uncomplaining, if not downright stoical! Thus, one can often hear phrases such as: 'I hope I'll be a good patient, nurse.' 'Can you *spare* just a minute, doctor?' 'If it's not too much *trouble*.' 'I hope I'm not making a *fuss*'.

However, the hospital environment is likely to intensify the patient's emotional vulnerability. There is a loss of independence, and even identity, which is made worse by shedding one's normal clothes and facing the world in night-clothes, which may themselves belong to the hospital. Each patient has to try to work out who is who in the hierarchy of the ward. It is akin to the feeling that most medical students feel on the first day *they* find themselves in a ward, uncertain of who the staff are and of the rules of the organization. In such a situation, every aspect of the environment begins to assume great importance and every communication is liable to be distorted by anxiety or the desire to conform. Even an innocent casual remark or gesture may be seized upon as something sinister.

At the same time, the patient is often exposed to potentially distressing operative or invasive procedures, necessary in the course of investigation or treatment. There is a tendency for the staff to play these down, skating over the discomfort, loss of dignity, or other distress they may cause. In such situations, patients can be helped by information of three types, well described by Wilson-Barnett [23]. These are: (1) procedural information, i.e. what will be done; (2) sensory information, i.e. what you will feel; (3) coping advice, i.e. how best you can cope.

The ward round

The main contact the patient has with the medical staff is usually during ward rounds. The patient is confronted with a group of people, rather than an individual. There is less privacy, and little intimacy. The encounter is likely to have an aura of protocol, rank, and formality. Often the inter- and intra-professional communication between doctor and nurse, and between consultant, registrar, house-officer, and student, takes precedence over unhurried sensitive communication with the patient. The group on the round is liable to cluster together near the foot of the bed, and the centre of interest may be more the case record, and the latest investigative reports, than the anxious and hesitant individual in the bed.

If, during a ward round the patient indicates a desire to talk, it is important that the senior person present should sit down close to the head of the bed and try to meet the need for unhurried 'private' conversation (Fig. 2.2). Sometimes it is impossible to achieve the appropriate degree of privacy and intimacy in an open ward; it is best then to talk with the patient again after the ward round is completed, in the privacy of a side room or office.

Apart from the time of history-taking on admission, two other important occasions when good communication is particularly important are (1) the completion of consent formalities, when

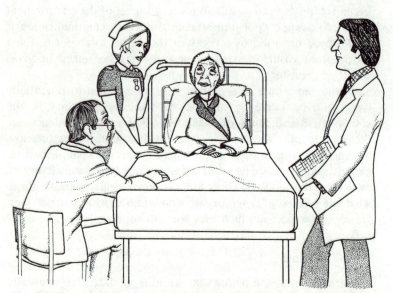

Fig. 2.2 Even during a busy ward round, the doctor must be ready to sit down and talk

adequate explanation is mandatory, and (2) the time of discharge from the ward, when good communication both with the patient and the general practitioner is crucial for continuity of care. Also be mindful, when consent is sought, of the pressure to conform which the patient is likely to feel in the strangeness of the ward environment.

Conducting an interview

Before considering the conduct of an interview in detail, it is useful to look at the elements involved in interpersonal communication. They include both verbal and non-verbal 'messages', which may be classified into four varieties.

(1) *verbal*: the choice of spoken words;

(2) *intonational*: the pitch, tone, or cadence of speech, the modulation of the voice; the whisper of confidentiality; the rising crescendo of anger or concern; the warm tones of interest and friendliness; the flat tones of despair;

(3) *paralinguistic*: non-verbal sound or utterances, e.g. the non-committal nasal 'hm-hm'; the sharp inspiration of surprise—'phew'; the expiratory puff signifying disgust;

(4) *kinesic*: communication through movements, facial expressions, posture or gesture—'body language'. (A clear, popular account of this aspect of communication may be found in Desmond Morris's *Manwatching* [24].)

While all these elements play a part in medical interviews, the learner should pay particular attention to body language, the unspoken messages conveyed without sound. In particular, he should be alert to any incongruity between what the patient is saying aloud and what his body is actually 'saying'. Tense knuckles, a furrowed brow, folded arms, or foot tapping, for example, may be conveying a message quite different from the patient's words. Emotion is conveyed more overtly by facial expression: this is normally symmetrical, but asymmetry can provide an indication that true feelings are being masked in some way. The student should never forget that his own body language is, in turn, communicating messages to the patient that may facilitate or inhibit communication between them. He should avoid, for example, folding his arms in a subconscious defensive posture, wielding the case folder prominently to convey his authority, or gazing at the case record when he should be looking at the patient's face. Communication can be greatly enhanced when verbal and non-verbal language are used synergistically, and incongruous messages are avoided.

Non-verbal communication is strengthened by the provision of comfort and privacy during an interview, by frequent but not intrusive eye contact, and by an open relaxed body posture with appropriate facial expressions and head movements. A distance between chairs which allows the doctor to reach out and touch the patient when this is appropriate is also helpful. In contrast, non-verbal communication is inhibited by lack of privacy or a noisy clinical environment, by infrequent eye contact, by folded arms or unfriendly facial expressions, or by ill-timed touch.

Some vocabulary of body language

Eye contact helps to convey interest and sincerity. Too intense eye contact can, however, be threatening and intimidatory. On occasion, it may elicit an aggressive response. Avoidance of eye contact can signal embarrassment, unreliability, or inattentiveness. A downcast gaze often signifies submissiveness, or occasionally sadness.

Much of the impact of first impressions is concerned with *facial expressions*. It is important that they are congruent with speech and speech content, or sincerity will not be conveyed.

Head posture and movements. The characteristic attitudes of talking heads, listening heads, and nods of agreement are very familiar. The head inclined to one side signifies a listening mode, and a degree of empathy.

Body movement and gestures. The emotions underlying words are often revealed in body movement. For example, a patient may describe a chest pain with clenched fists over the chest, or speak of difficulty in swallowing with a hand to the throat. Characteristic barrier signals which the doctor should avoid include crossing the arms or legs, and turning the head and body away from the speaker, signifying defensiveness, lack of interest, or even antipathy.

Often body language signalled by one individual induces the other to adopt similar 'mirror' gestures, indicating harmony with the speaker and agreement (gestural echoes). Feelings which cannot safely be shared with another may be expressed non-verbally despite the intention to conceal such thoughts. Examples of such leakage of concealed attitudes or information include feelings of impatience or desire to terminate the discussion, revealed by foot tapping, doodling, or other distracting finger movements. Similarly, increasing the distance between doctor and patient signals a wish for disengagement, or termination of the interview. Conversely, rapport can be facilitated by moving towards the patient, by leaning forward, or even by merely inclining the head towards the patient.

Touch and physical contact (see also Chapter 5). Physical contact, however trivial, can help to catalyse the sharing of feelings in a consultation. A handshake at the introduction and end of the interview can be all that is required to promote adequate rapport in a routine consultation. Inappropriate physical contact or ill-timed touching can be seen as shallow and patronizing, insincere, or threatening. But rapport is more frequently lost by the absence of physical contact than by its excessive use.

Intonation. The modulation of speech volume, intonation, and intervals of silence can convey much more than words themselves. When the manner and content of speech are incongruous, the non-verbal message is likely to be the more truthful. The patient who claims in flat mournful tones that he is feeling fine has to be considered to be low in mood until proved otherwise.

Reading and using body language, then, is essential for effective communication. With practice and experience, it can provide invaluable short-cuts to the growth of rapport. Remember that first impressions exchanged at the very start of the consultation can permanently influence the quality of the relationship. A warm friendly manner demonstrated by appropriate smiles and repeated eye contact signals readiness to communicate and a desire to help. A forward posture, open gestures, and positive head movements endorse this impression. A soft low volume voice with supportive vocalizations and positive use of silence all greatly facilitate the sharing of the patient's thoughts and feelings.

Some specific points about body language are emphasized in the next section, which considers in detail the conduct of an interview.

THE PHYSICAL SETTING

Communication can be helped or hindered by the physical setting in which the interview is being conducted. Normally, patient and doctor should be comfortably seated at the same level (Fig. 3.1). A possible exception to this arrangement might occur when the patient is sitting *higher* than the doctor, for example on the edge of the couch after physical examination has been completed (Fig. 3.2). If in bed, the patient should be encouraged to sit up wherever possible and made comfortable with pillow support, while the doctor draws up a chair alongside the bed (Fig. 2.2.).

The two chairs should usually be arranged about 1.5 metres apart, and set at an angle to each other, so that a direct face-to-face confrontation is avoided, but without a desk or other major piece of furniture intervening. In this position, the doctor and patient can easily make and break eye-to-eye contact, without any awkwardness. They are close enough to convey confidentiality, but not so close as to intrude upon each other's personal space. Exceptionally, it may be appropriate for the doctor to position his chair directly in front of a patient, for instance if he is speaking to

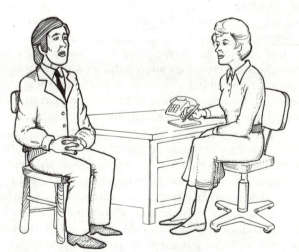

Fig. 3.1 Appropriate seating for good communication

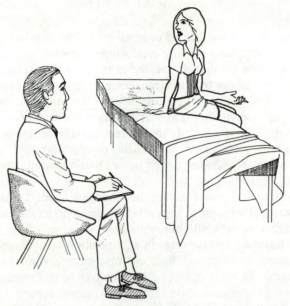

Fig. 3.2 The patient, sitting higher than the doctor, finds it easier to open up. (See also p. 153)

a very old person whose body movements are restricted, whose hearing is poor, or whose attention is impaired because of senile confusion or dementia.

The sort of interview arrangement that can have the most deleterious effects on communication is that in which the doctor faces the patient from behind a large desk piled with desk calendars, reference books, or even a vase of flowers, and beyond which the patient perches on a small plain chair, like a pupil in a headteacher's study (Fig. 3.3.).

Ideally, no one else should be present. If a nurse is in the room, she should have been clearly briefed to follow the conversation discreetly, and to leave the room if sensitive personal topics are raised or if the patient shows any hesitation in speaking to the doctor. A student or trainee, if present, should be introduced by name, and should sit near the doctor, but a little farther from the patient, within the same arc that the patient's chair is facing. From this position, the student can easily exchange eye-to-eye contact

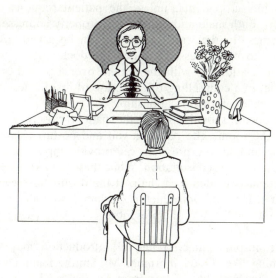

Fig. 3.3 The headmasterly 'I am in charge' setting: a grave barrier to communication

with patient and so participate in the interview, whether joining in the dialogue or not.

THE INTRODUCTION

At the outset, doctor and patient may sometimes be old acquaintances, but will often be complete strangers. When they are acquainted, their familiarity with each other socially may appear an obstacle to an effective therapeutic relationship, since a less clinical atmosphere obtains.

Modes of address

While it is appropriate to address a child by his or her first name, this may convey a patronizing air to an adult, especially an older or a disabled person, or might appear unduly familiar with a person of the opposite sex. It is therefore better to use formal names for out-patients, unless the patient requests otherwise. Muslims, both male and female, are properly addressed by their first names. In the ward, a patient can be asked 'How would you like to be addressed?' When the doctor needs to work in a closer relationship with the patient over a period of time, for example, in a counselling role, the use of first names can help to signal this less formal relationship.

The doctor should observe the patient closely as he or she enters the room. The patient's gait and posture, style of dress, manner, and facial expressions can provide important clues about the reason for the consultation. While these points are being noted, the patient is guided to a chair. If the doctor has never met the patient before, the introductory exchange should centre around 'Who are you?' before the presenting complaint ('How are you?') is discussed.

In a hospital clinic, a helpful introduction may be to say something like 'Good morning, Mr Smith. I am Dr Brown. I see you've brought a letter from Dr Green. Let me see what she has to tell me'. This allows the doctor a few moments to read through the letter of referral, while at the same time continuing to observe the patient's demeanour. As a prelude, if the complaint is not an urgent one, it can often be helpful to talk about the patient's general circumstances—occupation, age, marital status (and, if married, 'Have you a family?'). This initial exploration of 'Who are you?', suitably phrased in a friendly, open way, helps to put the patient at ease, provides the doctor with valuable background information, but also indicates to the patient from the outset that the doctor is concerned with him or her as a *person*, and is ready to talk about wider aspects of the patient's situation, not just the immediate complaint.

THE CORE OF THE INTERVIEW

After the introductory phase of the interview, the questions to be explored first can be phrased as:

(1) 'What is your problem?'

(2) 'How has it affected you?'

'*What is your problem?*' This question can be expressed in a number of ways, and the word 'problem' need not be used. 'What brings you to see me?' 'What can I do to help you?' 'What do you feel is wrong with yourself?' These are examples of how an open question can invite the patient to express what the trouble is. It is best to put aside one's pen as the question is asked.

Sometimes the patient has more than one problem and, while each should be noted, it may be necessary in the time available to concentrate on the immediate problem, or the main problem, and to plan a later interview to investigate other concerns the patient has mentioned. But whenever possible the patient should be given time at the initial interview to describe fully what his problems are. (See also p. 73).

One must be mindful, too, that the problem with which the patient presents may not in fact be the patient's real underlying problem. The patient may be using the presenting problem as a visiting card, a safe way of establishing contact to find out what sort of person the doctor is—how approachable, how understanding. Only then will the patient decide whether to reveal what the *real* problem is. For example, the teenager complaining of a mild vaginal discharge may in fact be anxious to discover whether she is pregnant, or whether she dare asks the doctor for contraceptive advice. The middle-aged man ostensibly complaining of tiredness or insomnia may be trying to pluck up courage so speak to the doctor about his erectile impotence. The patient with vague breathlessness may be too afraid to mention directly the lump she has felt in her breast.

The real problem is sometimes held back, and then slipped out just as the patient reaches the door, ready to leave.

'By the way, doctor, I've been a bit short of breath climbing the stairs recently. But I don't suppose that's anything serious, is it?'

'By the way, doctor, my daughter told me I ought to mention. I've got a small swelling down below. Sometime when you're not so busy, perhaps you could tell me what it is.'

For each complaint or problem, more detailed information should be sought, as Maguire and Rutter have described [25]. Accurate information, as far as this is possible, about the time of onset and the timing of subsequent developments and effects is usually of considerable diagnostic value. These details are set out more fully in the Appendix.

As well as obtaining an objective account of the sequence of events, it is often worthwhile eliciting the patient's subjective interpretation of the onset of the illness or problem: 'Did anything seem to start it off?', 'What seemed to start it off?', or (particularly if the disorder is not apparently due to organic disease) 'What do *you* think started it off?' Giving the patient the opportunity to express his views on the cause and nature of his indispositon can be valuable in preventing mistakes or misunderstandings, and often throws light on the diagnosis. This is especially relevant when the patient is from a different culture. (See also p. 214.) The verbal expressions and imagery used by a patient to describe symptoms can reveal something about how the illness is perceived and the degree of anxiety it has generated: 'The pain keeps gnawing away, as if it was eating into my bones.' 'I get these electric shock feelings in my head, and the top of my head prickles all over.' 'When the pain comes on, I feel absolutely lifeless. My whole body begins to go cold from the waist downwards.' One patient will dramatize his symptoms with evident exaggeration; another will display stoical indifference to his plight. Unexplained symptoms are more likely to be dismissed as due to psychological causes if described in graphic language, or with theatrical gestures.

When a complaint is of longer standing, or when the patient has apparently come to consult the doctor out of the blue, it is often revealing to enquire 'What made you decide to do something about it *now*?' In many instances, the patient's decision is triggered at some significant juncture in their life. Patients feel more vulnerable to illness following bereavement, for example, or when their ability to cope is overstretched by other stressful events. Sometimes, consultation is the result of intervention by a relative, or a response to a television programme highlighting a similar problem. Sometimes the alarm created by certain symptoms (such as bleeding or sharp pain) may have brought the patient. The motivation to consult, which can be unconscious, may not become apparent until the end of the consultation, or at a subsequent visit.

'*How has this affected you?*' '*How do you cope?*' An open question of this sort, introduced relatively early in the interview, is designed specifically to invite the patient to express his emotional response to the illness. Sometimes, an open question initially produces a non-committal response or a denial of affect from the patient. If so, a secondary and more specific enquiry later in the interview may help the patient respond, for example 'And how have you been feeling in yourself?' or 'How have you been able to cope?' or, more directly and empathically, 'You must have felt quite alarmed?'; or even, in certain situations, something like 'You must have been feeling at the end of your tether?'

Billings and Stoekle [26] have stressed that history-taking should regularly include an assessment of how patients understand their illness; what stress they experience; what coping mechanisms they adopt; what support they receive. This information is particularly important in serious stressful illness. The patient's strategies for coping may include pride in self-reliance; stoical religious faith; total reliance on the doctor; dependence on other family members; fatalistic acceptance.

Types of question

The sort of questions which have been suggested thus far to elicit from the patient a description of his complaint(s) are called *open questions*: 'What brings you to see me?' 'How has this affected you?' These questions do not presuppose a specific answer, but give the patient an open opportunity to respond in his own way, and in his own words. The more open the questions—'How did you feel about that?' 'What was your father like?'—the more revealing are the responses.

In contrast, *closed questions* require a specific answer. 'Is the pain worse on the left side or the right?' 'When did the dizziness begin?' 'How many times did you vomit?' 'Has any member of your family suffered from high blood-pressure?' These questions are interrogatory, and give the patient little room for explanation or qualification, particularly if they follow in quick succession. They are often more taxing to answer precisely, especially if the patient is frail, forgetful, or in pain.

A third type of question is the *leading question*, favoured by barristers because it is framed in such a way as to almost invite a particular answer. 'Would you say you usually get loose motions after eating very spicy food?' 'And did you notice that your urine became a little darker in colour after the pain came on?' Leading questions are best avoided when the patient is initially trying to describe his symptoms, since they may bias the replies. But with experience, leading questions *can* be used to advantage later in an interview to confirm a diagnostic hunch: 'So it sounds as if these blackouts come on only when you are looking up above your head?' or to help put into words something the patient may be finding difficult to say: 'Would you say that your husband's attitude/daughter's behaviour makes you feel very angry inside?'

In contrast to leading questions, which can be only too easy to answer, questions beginning 'Why . . .?' are often difficult to answer, and may readily sound critical or inquisitorial. In general, they are best avoided.

MODELS OF DIAGNOSTIC REASONING

'Systematic' interviewing: a bad model

At this stage in the history, having heard the patient's account of the presenting complaint or problem, the student or inexperienced doctor thereafter may tend to follow a predetermined outline for the rest of the interview. This is generally based on a sequence of headings, covering the full content of a comprehensive history, i.e. a review of the function of the main organ systems; past medical history; family history; social history. Because he has been taught what a complete medical history can encompass, a learner may be at pains to ensure that every area is covered systematically and that no detail of possible importance is omitted (see Appendix).

The unfortunate temptation is that, by following a structured pattern through the interview, the student may feel a greater sense of confidence. Most students are anxious when they first embark upon solo interviews with patients. They may be afraid that they could lose control of the interview, or forget what to ask next and therefore 'dry up'. In the back of their minds is a fairly long checklist of questions, which they tend to work through steadily.

This approach (Fig. 3.4), which can easily become a habit, tends regrettably to result in a structured interrogation of the patient, who is expected to answer a long succession of direct, closed questions. These may appear to the patient to have little or no relevance to his immediate complaints. A doctor-led agenda, trawling for a diagnosis, can leave the patient's problems and

---

1. Comprehensive systematic history-taking

　　　then

2. Systematic clinical examination

　　　then

3. A wide range of potentially relevant investigations

　　　then

4. Diagnostic reasoning based on all the above information

Fig. 3.4 Model of the 'systematic' approach to diagnosis

concerns at risk of being sidelined or overlooked altogether. If the interviewer adopts an interrogatory style from the very beginning, tightly controlling the sequence of question and answer, anxious not to lose the thread as he ploughs through his checklist of topics, the patient is unlikely to have adequate opportunity to express his problems. The style of the interview will stifle expression of the affective aspects of the patient's illness.

If any direct questioning of a systematic nature has to be included in a consultation, a guiding principle is that such questions should be tagged on only in the latter part of the interview, after the patient has been given every chance to respond to more open questions in his own words.

MORE EFFICIENT MODELS OF
DIAGNOSTIC REASONING

The systematic, comprehensive model of history-taking and clinical examination referred to above has traditionally been taught to students in hospital as part of their initiation into clinical work. Every student, of course, needs to become familiar with the language of all aspects of history-taking, and with a great variety of normal as well as abnormal physical findings. For this purpose, unselective comprehensive enquiries and systematic examination provide repeated basic practice.

But they inculcate a bad model for communication. This approach to diagnosis is certainly not adopted during consultation by experienced clinicians. The blunderbuss approach with a full detailed history, top-to-toe clinical examination, and a battery of all potentially relevant investigations has to be replaced by more efficient methods. Furthermore, experience brings an awareness that diagnosis is not an end in itself (apart from the intellectual self-satisfaction it may afford). Diagnosis is, in effect, a statement of probability which forms the basis on which decisions about management are made. In these practical terms, a satisfactory diagnosis does not have to be absolutely certain. However, the assumed diagnosis must ensure that the patient will be better managed on the basis of that assumption rather than on any alternative conclusion. Macartney [27] emphasized and illustrated this point very clearly. To quote Kassirer's incisive paper titled 'Our stubborn quest for diagnostic certainty: a cause of excessive testing' [28]: 'Absolute certainty in diagnosis is unattainable, no matter how much information we gather, how many observations we make, or how many tests we perform. A diagnosis is a hypothesis about the nature of a patient's illness, derived from observations by the use of inference. Our confidence in a given diagnosis is enhanced by data that either favour it, or argue against other competing hypotheses. More tests do not necessarily produce more certainty, but may merely initiate a cascade of more hazardous tests'.

Review of the pattern of working of skilled and experienced doctors has allowed their methods of history-taking and diagnostic reasoning to be analysed in some detail [29,30,31]. The patterns revealed are quite different from the systematic model described above and illustrated schematically in Fig. 3.4. Interpersonal skills, reasoning skills, and clinical examination skills are all involved. Various attempts have been made to delineate and explain the stages and steps which may be involved in diagnostic reasoning. Of the different 'models' of diagnostic logic which can be formulated, the following are now well recognized.

The hypothetico-deductive model

Clinicians who view medicine as Science are pleased to invest their diagnostic reasoning with a scientific aura. According to this model, the diagnostic process begins by collecting observations

1. Eliciting the presenting complaints

   then

2. Forming a number of diagnostic hypotheses

   then

3. Seeking to validate or negate these hypotheses by
   selective questioning
   selective physical examination
   selective investigations

Fig. 3.5 Model of the hypothetico-deductive approach to diagnosis

about the patient (from the history and initial examination). From these observations, the clinician generates a number of diagnostic hypotheses (usually not more than four or five) to explain the observations made. These hypotheses can spring from the doctor's experience, hunch, or even intuition [33,33]. He then seeks to eliminate or reinforce the various possibilities by further observations, tests, and investigations. In this model, the generation and testing of hypotheses is seen as the scientific 'core' of diagnostic reasoning (Fig. 3.5).

If the clinician aims for Scientific thinking, he should understand that scientific hypotheses can never be proven; testing may show hypotheses to be false, but can never provide absolute certainty of their truth.

Diagnostic algorithms

The notion underlying a diagnostic algorithm is in essence the flowchart adopted in certain types of digital computer programs. With its aid, a decision-tree can be created, leading by alternative pathways towards different diagnoses. Figures 3.6 and 3.7 are examples of diagnostic algorithms published in the *British Medical Journal* (reproduced by permission of the editor and authors).

This analytical model allows an economy of reasoning and an apparent precision of diagnosis that is very attractive but that is just not possible in many cases. However, algorithms can sometimes provide clear guidelines for dealing with particular

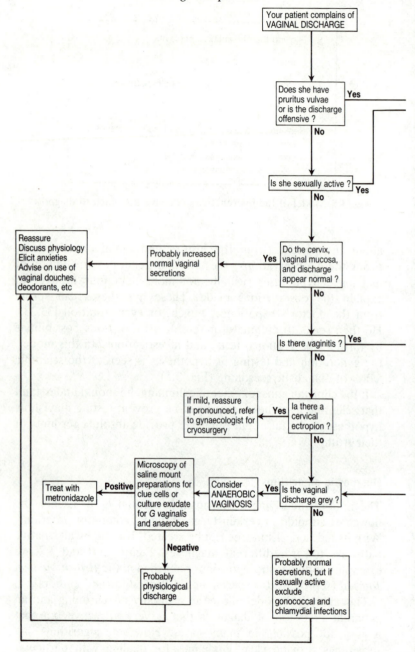

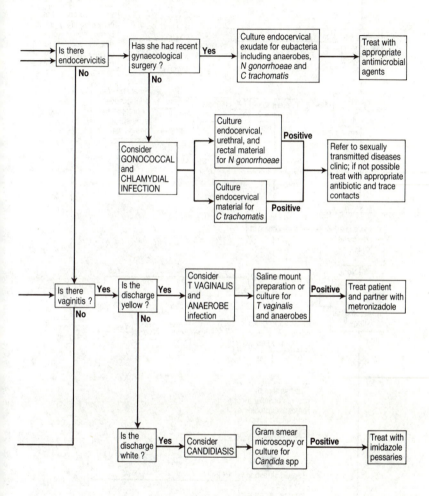

Fig. 3.6 Example of a diagnostic algorithm, outlining the diagnosis of vaginal discharge. (Reproduced from the *British Medical Journal* by kind permission)

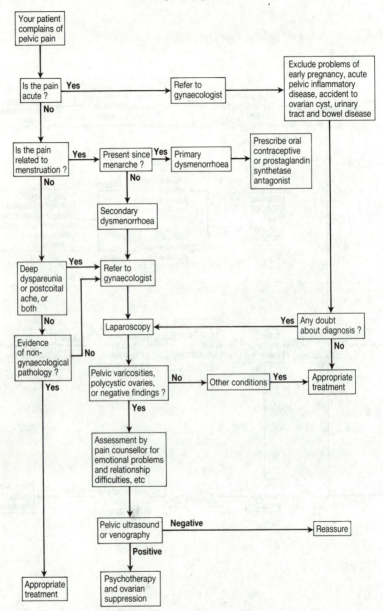

Fig. 3.7 Example of a diagnostic algorithm, outlining the diagnosis of pelvic pain. (Reproduced from the *British Medical Journal* by kind permission)

clinical problems, and so help the learner to adopt some of the skills of the expert.

The probabilistic model (Bayes' theorem)

The theorem of Bayes (which few clinicians have studied, and even fewer fully understood!) calculates the probability of a future event on the basis of prior probabilities of associated past events. In the diagnostic context, Bayesian analysis allows the probabilities of different diagnoses in a particular patient to be calculated (and therefore ranked) from the known features of the clinical presentation of other patients previously evaluated. The validity of this model has been clearly demonstrated by its successful application in computer programs for the elucidation of everyday diagnostic problems, such as the diagnosis of abdominal pain [34,35] and of congenital heart disease [36].

The basic requirement for *precise* application of Bayes' theorem is a bank of data that can be represented as a conditional probability matrix, of which Fig. 3.8 is a notional example relating to some of the features present in a supposed population of patients complaining of vaginal discharge. From such a tabulation, using Bayes' theorem, the probability of each diagnosis could be calculated for an individual patient with a particular combination of symptoms.

In day-to-day practice, clinicians do not, of course, engage in mathematical computation in this precise way unless they are indeed using a suitably programmed computer, but often the pattern of their diagnostic reasoning follows a Bayesian model. They have accumulated from past experience a mental databank

	Trichomonas	Thrush	Anaerobic vaginitis	Gonorrhoea	Chlamydia
Yellow discharge	74	12	42	27	24
Itching	86	95	2	2	4
Odour	94	3	97	4	5
Dyspareunia	62	88	5	6	7

Fig. 3.8 Percentage frequency (notional) of certain symptoms associated with various causes of vaginal discharge

1. Eliciting the presenting complaints
then
2. Forming a short list of probable diagnoses, based on the doctor's knowledge of clinical epidemiology
then
3. Eliciting futher clinical information selectively, to refine the estimate of diagnostic probabilities

Fig. 3.9 Model of the probabilistic (Bayesian) approach to diagnosis

of impressions, correlating certain clinical findings with particular diagnoses, with greater or lesser probability. They selectively elicit information about those parameters they have found to have the greatest discriminatory power. In this way, they mentally juggle with a league-table of probable diagnoses [33] (Fig. 3.9). Using the same example as in Fig. 3.8, if a patient complains of vaginal discharge, the doctor will have several possibilities in mind. The discharge is described as yellow: thrush infection seems a low probability. Is dyspareunia (painful intercourse) present? No: thrush infection is therefore doubly unlikely. Is the discharge malodorous? Yes: trichomonal infection or anaerobic infection are now emerging as the most probable diagnoses. Is there itching? No: anaerobic vaginitis thus emerges as the most likely cause of the patient's symptoms on the basis of the selective enquiries made. Confirmatory tests (microscopy for 'clue' cells, amine test) could put the matter beyond reasonable doubt.

Cluster recognition: syndromes

In certain illnesses, a characteristic and sometimes virtually unique cluster of symptoms and/or signs occurs. Just as an ornithologist can recognize a particular bird from a brief glimpse of three or four features—its wing action, a flash of throat colour, its length of tail, and favoured place of concealment—so an experienced clinician can sometimes spot a diagnosis in a few moments. The less common the syndrome, and the more unusual the associated signs and symptoms, the more pathognomonic the conclusion becomes. With widening clinical knowledge, the experienced clinician can occasionally adopt this sort of diagnostic short cut to great effect.

Common elements

The distinctive labels attached to different models of diagnostic reasoning obscure recognition of their essentially common elements. They all involve information-gathering, usually more and more selectively as the history unfolds. These observations are then evaluated and interpreted by a process of reasoning which is not always confined to the frame of logic of a single model, but which often includes elements from all the patterns of reasoning mentioned above. The tentative diagnostic inferences are then tested by further selective enquiries, clinical examination, and investigative procedures.

FUNCTIONAL DISORDERS

The models of diagnostic logic described above are all generally applicable to patients whose complaints arise from an organic cause. The pathways of diagnostic reasoning seek to trace the symptoms back to their origins, and identify their aetiology in terms of physico-chemical mechanisms.

However, in many other patients, organic disease is not the cause of the symptoms, particularly those patients with chronic, recurrent, or ill-defined complaints (such as vague abdominal pain, headaches, breathlessness, dizziness, irritability, impaired concentration, inability to cope) or with mood disturbances (feeling anxious or depressed). Such disorders are variously described as functional or psychosomatic, and their origin is likely to be related to some focus of emotional stress. This may centre around an aspect of the patient's external environment—unemployment, fear of redundancy, overwork, other occupational stress, bad housing, vandalism or burglary, overcrowding, homelessness; around strained interpersonal relationships, especially those with close family members; or around unresolved emotional conflict within the patient's inner self. Sometimes, traumatic events have occurred much earlier in life—separation from parents, being jilted, bereavement, sexual assault/abuse, divorce, unsuccessful pregnancy.

To recognize functional disorders, we need to maintain a sensitive awareness with every patient of the close interaction of mind and body in the aetiology as well as the sequelae of ill health. In practical terms, it is essential to use the time available to find out as much as possible about the patient's life and circumstances, past and present (see also p. 97).

Additional time is required to gather the information necessary to fill in this wider view of the patient. Whenever possible, multiple interviews will allow better exploration of the patient's circumstances and relationships in an unpressured open pattern of dialogue. This makes it easier for a hesitant patient to disclose things that might be troubling him, and affords greater opportunity for the doctor to divert in response to clues or cues. Again, if counselling (see p. 123) is needed to help the patient to resolve some or all of his difficulties, this too will necessitate longer interviewing sessions.

This broader view of the patient, required to identify and understand the nature of his illness, is sometimes labelled 'holistic', and can be contrasted with the reductionist analysis of disease processes in physico-chemical terms. But the antithesis is a false one. These are not necessarily alternative, but rather complementary views of the patient, and each is incomplete and inadequate by itself. Just as the revealing tones of white light can only arise from the blending of different wavelengths of coloured light across the span of the visible spectrum, so information of widely differing modalities is required to delineate a true perspective of the patient. Even when an illness is conclusively organic in origin, there are invariably repercussions affecting many aspects of the patient's life, and not least his emotions and his relationships with others. In addition, a considerable number of common disorders with organic manifestations, such as asthma, irritable bowel syndrome, ulcerative colitis, migraine, and eczema, are stress-related, so that again the widest information about the patient is likely to be of relevance.

Psychosomatic (functional) illness is given more detailed consideration in Chapter 9.

DOVE-TAILING THE HISTORY TAKING AND CLINICAL EXAMINATION

In practice, the history-taking and clinical examination are generally not separate consecutive parts of the consultation; they proceed alongside each other as complementary parts of the process of diagnostic reasoning. Although the patients' consent to examination can often be inferred, it will usually promote trust if consent is asked for 'May I examine you now?' This seeking and giving of consent has particular value in the case of a child patient, or a female from a conservative culture.

The degree of overlap between history-taking and examination is considerably influenced by the nature and site of the patient's complaint. If, for example, the patient complains of a sore eye, or a painful toe, or a skin eruption on the hands, the doctor will want to begin examining the affected part early in the consultation. If, on the other hand, it is clear from the nature of the presenting symptoms that the patient will have to undress completely for a more comprehensive examination, the doctor will probably prefer to proceed as far as possible with his diagnostic questioning before asking the patient to undress.

Even if the doctor feels he has completed the formal history-taking before he embarks on the physical examination, he should nevertheless continue to communicate sensitively during the examination itself. If either patient or doctor feels awkward with the intimacy attending undressing and physical examination, this is likely to create an obstacle to continuing communication. Initially, then, the patient should be told clearly how much undressing is necessary—what to take off, and perhaps what to leave on. 'I'd like you to take off everything except your under-pants.' 'Please take off your shoes, tights and pants so that I can examine you.'

In this situation, the learner has to avoid adopting an exaggerated and distant formality, in which the silence is broken only by an occasional curt instruction: 'Take a deep breath.' 'Again.' However, attempts to overcome awkwardness with a stream of distracting social chit-chat about irrelevant topics such as the weather, or holidays, are not helpful. To avoid a silence, which would be both embarrassing and probably alarming, the patient could be asked, for example, more detailed questions about his job, or a parent could be asked about his or her children. If through professional skill a comfortable sense of relaxed intimacy is created during the physical examination, the patient will be more willing to voice worrying or delicate concerns.

It is helpful to explain to the patient what you are about to do *before* you do it, and this is especially important if the patient cannot easily see what is happening. This applies, for instance, when firm palpation or percussion over the spine is to be performed, or when, with the patient in the left lateral position, rectal examination is to be undertaken. Particularly during physical examination, the doctor should choose simple words and phrases that the patient can easily understand and that will not cause alarm or embarrassment. During clinical examination, the patient's anxiety about what the doctor is perhaps going to discover can be quite intense, and questions can readily acquire a threatening implication. For example, a patient could be caused alarm if she were asked during auscultation of the heart whether there was a family history of heart disease, or if, during vaginal examination, she was suddenly asked 'How long is it since you had a cervical smear?' In each instance, the patient might well jump to the conclusion that the doctor had found something ominous.

SELECTIVE BUT SENSITIVE ENQUIRIES

At the beginning of the interview the initiative is with the patient and the doctor is mainly an observant listener, but as the consultation proceeds the initiative moves to the doctor, who has to direct his questions more selectively and searchingly as the process of diagnosis advances, trying to ensure that the information elicited is accurate.

But although the doctor is very much in the driving seat during the heart of the consultation, the open and sensitive patient-centred approach taken during the initial unfolding of the presenting problem is still required. The quest for accurate information should not be tinged with irritability because some patients give vague or inconsistent replies. The manner and content of the patient's responses to these selective questions may provide an indication of the patient's feelings, which the doctor should be alert to recognize, responding appropriately. The degree of openness with which questions are posed can help or hinder the expression of feeling. For example, it is often helpful to ask 'Have you always enjoyed good health?' rather than 'What previous illnesses or operations have you had?' Answers to the first question are more likely to reveal something of patients' attitudes towards their general health. Similarly, it is better to ask 'Do the members of your family all enjoy good health?' rather than asking only about particular diseases.

CONCLUDING THE HISTORY-TAKING

Before concluding the history-taking, it is often worth while to pose a further open question such as 'Well, have we covered all aspects of the problem?' or 'Have you anything more you want to tell me?' This helps to ensure that patients who have been slow to respond earlier in the interview, or who may have forgotten something regarded as important, have another opportunity to state what is on their mind. It can be particularly important when interviewing an anxious or elderly, forgetful person.

THE VALUE OF EXPERIENCE

The application of all forms of diagnostic reasoning in a selective but reliable way depends crucially upon a good knowledge of the natural history of disease, and especially of the manner in which it presents. Such knowledge is an essential element in all the diagnostic models reviewed above. It may be structured as an algorithm; it may involve pattern recognition—the significance of particular clusters of clinical features; or it may provide the basis of a statistical assessment of probabilities in the circumstances of a particular case. As the student's knowledge of medicine grows and the diagnostic logic at his disposal is refined, redundant steps in the diagnostic process can be avoided. The whole procedure of consultation becomes quicker, more efficient, and more cost-effective as superfluous diagnostic enquiries and investigations are eliminated. This is why time spent in the clinic, consulting room, or ward listening carefully to patients' accounts of their illnesses, offers the student learning experiences of enormous value.

However, diagnosis cannot always be reached by the sort of

elegant definitive analysis provided by some of the above models. Students should not be discouraged if sometimes they have just to gather *all* the information they can about the patient and then plan a relatively wide range of investigations.

Life events

With increasing experience, a doctor comes to understand more about not only the natural history of disease but also the way in which people tend to react to health problems. He begins to recognize that patients react not only to their own illnesses but also to those of other family members, friends, and neighbours. For example, the death of a parent or close sibling during childhood may leave a legacy of insecurity or depression; the fact that her mother had a hysterectomy may leave a patient with a niggling worry that the same thing will happen to her; breast cancer in a friend or neighbour may trigger off the anxiety underlying a patient's present complaints.

Anxiety about health is not only precipitated by contact with, or the threat of illness. The underlying emotional tension which has provoked the patient's complaint may relate to another area of the patient's life: the threat of redundancy; the stress of promotion or a new job; the imminence of marriage, or an examination; the anniversary of a bereavement.

Flexible responses essential

So far, we have attempted to set out some sort of outline for history-taking, intended to facilitate good communication between patient and doctor and, in particular, to provide clear opportunities for the patient to speak about attitudes and feelings surrounding the illness. The following basic elements have been identified.

- A comfortable, supportive physical setting.

- A warm introduction, to elicit a response to 'Who are you?'

- An open initial enquiry, allowing the patient every opportunity to present the problem in his or her own words.

- A specific invitation to describe any affective responses to illness.

- A sequence of selective questions in the search for a diagnosis, usually supplemented by initial clinical examination.

- Sometimes, in the latter part of an interview in the hospital setting, some systematic questioning to provide a comprehensive overview of the patient.

- Further 'open' questions.

This outline is inadequate in one important respect. No individual interview, with its exploration of a particular patient's problem(s), can be expected to follow a predetermined pattern. Unexpected information may begin to emerge, and the patient may react in an unexpected way to certain questions, providing verbal or non-verbal clues.

A medical interview, therefore, should not be planned in a rigid formulaic way with a set structure. An essential feature is the responsiveness of the doctor (see p. 65) and his awareness that at any point the patient might reveal a clue, or drop a cue that the doctor must be ready to recognize and respond to, branching away from the intended pattern of the interview to follow a different line of enquiry. Such responsiveness is discussed in more detail in Chapter 6.

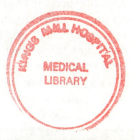

Facilitating communication

4

After reviewing the broad strategy of the interview, we need to look at the tactics of the dialogue. Of particular importance are the methods by which a doctor can facilitate communication. These help to elicit as accurately as possible, in the limited time available, the information needed to make a diagnosis and plan treatment, while giving the patient adequate opportunity to express his feelings. Whatever the nature of the verbal exchanges, the patient's body language, which is likely to convey information of its own, must be carefully observed throughout.

VOCABULARY

The doctor should ask questions in clear, unambiguous language suitable to the patient's age, education, and cultural background; the information often gained during the introductory phase of the interview about the patient's general background will be of assistance. Unsuitable language, whether in vocabulary, accent, or overformal style, can regrettably inhibit rather than facilitate dialogue. The vocabulary chosen should not include technical terms or unfamiliar words. If the doctor senses that the patient is hesitating for want of suitable vocabulary, he should attempt to include the needed non-technical words in his questions. This applies especially to enquiries about potentially embarrassing topics such as excretory or sexual function. When the doctor supplies in a comfortable, open way suitable simple but explicit words describing these functions, this does more to facilitate discussion than merely providing a vocabulary.

The patient can follow the purpose and direction of the doctor's enquiries more readily if the pattern of questions follows some logical grouping and sequence. If the doctor does have an after-thought, he should explain himself; he might say for example 'Now could we just go back to this question of your indigestion? Was there ever an occasion when food actually seemed to stick in your throat?'

Topics that the patient may feel sensitive about should usually be introduced in the latter part of an interview, when confidence and rapport have been established. Again, they should wherever possible form part of a logical sequence of related enquiries. For example, questions about urinary or faecal incontinence should follow enquiries about normal excretory function, and questions about dyspareunia (painful intercourse) can follow those about other types of pelvic pain, pruritus vulvae, or similar pelvic complaints.

Not all patients are reluctant to speak frankly and freely to a doctor. Some may be so ready to talk that the doctor's problem is to control their garrulous chatter. However, much greater skill is required to help a hesitant patient open up.

CAUSES OF RETICENCE

It is first all-important to try to recognize *why* a patient is holding back or having difficulty in expressing himself freely, so that whenever possible something can be done about the inhibiting factor(s). The patient's reticence may be due to the following.

- The presence of a third party: a nurse, a student, or even an accompanying relative. They should, if necessary, be asked tactfully to leave the room.

- Sometimes the fact that the doctor is also the family doctor may inhibit an adolescent from speaking freely.

- The patient may fear that revealing his complaints will lead to the realization of his worst fears: a diagnosis of serious disease, admission to hospital, an operation.

- A reluctance to take up the doctor's time with concerns that the patient may feel are undeserving of his time and attention: 'You are always a very busy man, doctor, and there are several folk still waiting to see you.'

- Embarrassment or shame about the nature of the complaint. This might apply to a wide range of disorders, but especially to those with a sexual association: venereal disease; other genital complaints; drinking problems; pregnancy in the unmarried, widowed, or separated; impotence.

- Cultural barriers. For example, many Asian women find it difficult to discuss personal or marital problems with a male doctor or even with a strange female doctor. A youthful or a venerable-looking doctor may be seen as an unsuitable confidant if he or she obviously belongs to a different generation from the patient.

These are some of the more specific obstacles to open communication that should be kept in mind if a patient is holding back. With experience and training, the student will learn to recognize the causes of reticence and be able to overcome them. The communication skills to be employed include non-verbal (body) language, speech, and appropriate use of silences.

WAYS OF FACILITATING COMMUNICATION

Non-verbal

An unhurried manner is basic essential, conveying the message 'I have time to listen'. While listening, the doctor can nod attentively (but not nod off!). He should not be afraid to smile, since smiling is often the best way of conveying reassurance, understanding, acceptance, and warmth. If the patient pauses, the doctor may lower his eyes for a moment without looking away and then look back at the patient's face, signalling 'Go on'. At certain points, it is helpful to discard pen and notes in an obvious way, and push them to one side, perhaps adding 'So tell me more about . . .', referring to a rather sensitive topic that has not yet been ventilated adequately, and about which the doctor feels there is more to be said. If what seems a delicate question has to be posed, it can help to lean forward towards the patient, underlining the intimacy and confidentiality of the conversation.

As the patient talks, the doctor is not just a passive observer, but is 'actively' listening—using appropriate body language; hearing not only what the patient says, but how he says it; noting the tone of his voice, his choice of words, expressions, and gestures. Appropriate use of touch can help to convey concern, reassurance, and encouragement, particularly when dealing with the frail, the fearful, or depressed. A brief contact on the back of the hand or forearm (which are the least threatening areas) will often be enough. The gentleness used during clinical touching will also convey a message (p.53).

By speech

A variety of simple short responses from the doctor will encourage the patient to continue speaking, especially if accompanied by a brief smile: 'Yes, I see', 'Go on', 'I understand', or sometimes 'I don't quite follow you', inviting the patient to give a fuller account.

Reflecting

Somewhat similarly, but more positively, the doctor can encourage the patient to continue speaking by repeating, and so *reflecting* back to him, a phrase, idea, or significant word from what the patient has just said. By picking up a word or expression in this way, the patient is prompted to express himself further.

Here is an example of this technique of reflecting.

'Doctor, I can always sense when my husband is building up towards another bout of heavy drinking, but . . . well . . . I just feel there's absolutely *nothing* I can do about it. I've given up.'
'Nothing?'
'Well . . . maybe . . . You see, I'm always afraid if I say anything that I'll be to blame for what he's doing. Do you think I should try to talk to him?'

Another example might be the following interchange.

'The period pains are not too bad, but the headaches I get before the period starts to make me *desperately* miserable for three or four days every month.'
'You feel desperate at that time?'
'Yes, to be honest, I do. Recently there have been several times when I've thought of doing away with myself, because at the time it felt as if there was nothing to live for.'

Clarifying

This term is used to describe another ploy which helps to make clear to the patient what he is trying to put into words, and also allows the doctor to check on his own tentative deductions:

'You seem to be saying that, since the pains began, you not only gradually lost your appetite, but also lost interest in all kinds of everyday activities. Is that correct?'

Or, to offer another example:

'Are you trying to tell me that you're really afraid this is something very serious? Is that what you feel?'

Summarizing

It can also be very helpful, particularly when the history is long and complicated, to attempt at some point to summarize all or part of the patient's account of things. This recapitulation must be done tentatively, getting the patient to corroborate the more important details. Otherwise there is the danger that a compliant patient may just accept the doctor's version of the history, which could reflect more the doctor's preconceived ideas than what actually happened:

'So if we could just go over the main points of what you have told me so far. Your periods were perfectly normal and regular until five months ago. Then you missed two periods completely, and then bled heavily for three weeks. Since that time there has been some scanty loss most days, but no pain at any time. Is that correct?'

'Could we just recap to be sure I have got it right? You had just finished a huge Chinese take-away, when you suddenly began to perspire. When you got up to open the window, the pain behind your breastbone began, and your knees gave way. When you came to on the floor, you felt very nauseated, and were seeing double for a time, and you had this big cut on your forehead.'

By appropriate use of silences

One of the nightmarish anxieties of the inexperienced student or doctor is that he will dry up during the interview; that he will run out of questions; and that an embarrassing silence will open up, creating discomfort and disrupting communication. In contrast, an easy interview often seems to flow along in sustained dialogue with barely a pause. The learner can avoid an undesirable hiatus of his own making by having in reserve one or two fill-in questions that cannot be answered very briefly (e.g. a question about the patient's childhood or about other family members) but which have some loose relevance to the presenting symptoms. One of these questions can be thrown in when such a silence threatens; while the patient is answering, the questioner can pick up the threads and poise himself for his next line of enquiry.

It is a mistake to believe that silences must be avoided at all costs. Apart from the nervous silences of the beginner referred to above, other silences can occur, when the patient runs out of words or is unsure about expressing his feelings. In this situation, the doctor must resist the temptation to disarm the silence promptly with a new question on a new topic, and so thereby suppress what the patient may be struggling to say. Rather, he should deliberately let the silence remain unbroken for a little time, while continuing to look at the patient with a facial expression of unhurried interest and concern. Then he can signal 'Go on' either verbally or non-verbally.

FACILITATING THE OPEN EXPRESSION OF DEEP FEELINGS; MIRRORING AND CONFRONTATION

An interview in which the patient 'gets upset' is generally thought of as undesirable. Indeed, the very idea that the patient might burst into tears or erupt in anger would provide many inexperienced doctors with feelings of discomfort and embarrassment, or a sense of failure. (Their response to tears resembles their reaction to haemorrhage—get it stopped as quickly as possible!)

The same inhibitions about expressing emotions in the course of a formal professional consultation affect patients no less than doctors—'I'm sorry I got upset just now.' 'I shouldn't have let myself go like that—I feel ashamed.' 'I didn't want my feelings to get the better of me. I'd promised myself I wouldn't let that happen.' So, even when patients are experiencing strong feelings that are flooding up below the surface, they are likely to make every effort to restrain or conceal them, whereas the expression of the distressing feelings—the catharsis—may be an important part of the therapeutic value of the interview.

Hence, if the patient shows evidence of suppressed emotion, for example if tears begin to well up, the doctor must resist the temptation to jump in with distracting questions on a less emotive topic. He most certainly should not exhort such patients to cheer up, or to 'take a grip on themselves'.

As a first response to evidence of emotion, it is best if the doctor remains silent for a moment to allow the patient to stay with the feelings; to 'bridge' the silence the doctor should continue to look towards the patient with an expression of concern.

Mirroring

The patient is usually helped to put his feelings into words if the doctor acts as a sort of mirror in which the patient's feelings are revealed. The doctor might quietly say (for example), 'Your eyes began to water when you spoke about that' or 'You appeared a bit upset even mentioning your son.'

Confrontation

In some instances, the doctor can help the expression of feelings by confronting the patient directly, though quietly and sympathetically, with the emotions he is observing: 'You look very angry', 'You seem very upset just now', or 'You look as though you are going to cry.' Such remarks seek to identify the patient's feelings and give permission for their open acknowledgement, which is then likely to follow with therapeutic benefit. The essential first step in coming to terms with any distressing emotion whether it be grief, anger, fear, or some other painful feeling, is to acknowledge it, rather than to deny or suppress it.

This confronting of the patient with the reality of his feelings should be based on what the doctor actually observes, and not upon inferences or interpretations. The identification of the feelings helps to convey that the doctor understands how the patient is feeling. The essence of successful confrontation is that, when it is appropriately timed, the patient's suppressed feelings cannot be denied expression.

INCONGRUOUS ELEMENTS WITHIN
THE INTERVIEW

In drawing together some of what has been learnt about conducting an interview, it can be seen that there are incongruous activities and that skill is needed to maintain the most effective balance between them. Table 4.1 sets out these pairs of contrasting activities.

Table 4.1 Incongruous elements within the interview

Facilitating communication	Controlling the interview
Listening in an unhurried way	Covering all relevant enquiries adequately in the limited time available
Avoiding inhibiting the patient	Keeping the patient to the point
Seeking accurate information about illness	Tolerating vagueness, especially from the elderly and the anxious
Endeavouring to follow a diagnostic pathway of enquiries	Being ready to divert and respond to the patient's disclosures and cues
Keeping a full, accurate record of the interview	Not allowing the pen and notes to inhibit free communication

5 Communication by and during touching

Discussion of interpersonal communication would not be complete without reference to communication by touching. In all cultures, touching is a basic form of both social and sexual communication. Lovers touch to convey affection, and so do all human beings when they wish to convey, without the use of words, affinity and warmth, sympathy, encouragement, or reassurance. When comforting a patient in pain, a hand instinctively reaches out to touch. In the labour room, for example, one may quietly stroke the patient's arm or her hair during painful contractions. I have sometimes noticed in dealing with demented old ladies, agitated almost beyond the reach of words, that gentle facial stroking can help to reassure and calm them, allowing some communication to be established.

Here, though, we are primarily considering touching as a professional skill, routine clinical palpation, by which a doctor explores the surfaces of patients' bodies and the intimacies of their various orifices, including the erogenous zones, as a regular element of everyday work. What significance does this have in the communication process?

CLINICAL EXAMINATION WORLD-WIDE

The routine touching of clinical examination is not a universal of medicine world-wide, but is particularly a feature of allopathic medicine within (say) the last 400 years and particularly the last 200 years. After the Renaissance, the expanding study of anatomy, pathology, and physiology began to provide the evidence on which, during the 19th century, a more rational, analytical and secular system of medical practice could be based. In this, clinical examination for the first time provided important diagnostic information.

In many of the systems of traditional medicine world-wide—
Ayurvedic, Unani, African traditional, and so on—physical examination, apart perhaps from feeling the pulse or inspecting the
tongue and urine, plays little or no part, and the pattern of communication between practitioner and patient reflects this absence
of physical intimacy.

It is an interesting speculation that the increasing sophistication
of the biochemical analysis of blood, urine, and other body fluids,
together with the expansion of ultrasonic and isotope imaging,
magnetic resonance imaging, and computer-assisted tomography,
not to mention interventional and conventional radiology and a
growing range of other investigative techniques, may well be leading to clinical practice in which conventional physical examination
will be minimal, or may even become extinct!

THE NEED TO MAKE TOUCHING SAFE

It has already been pointed out that doctors require a protective
mechanism to professionalize the intimacy that is inseparable from
clinical examination, and that they may achieve this only by virtually excluding the patient's sexuality from thought or discussion
and by eliminating warmth within the professional relationship.
Psychiatrists, in contrast, who are accustomed to exploring verbally
the intimacies of patients' personal and sexual relationships, are
usually reluctant to carry out personally a physical examination of
the same individuals.

How, then, do the sexual connotations of touching influence
the doctor's professional touching and the part this plays in communication? For example, there is an obvious contrast between
doctors' style when examining a child as compared with an
adult. A paediatric textbook will describe clearly how to obtain
the maximum information from abdominal palpation of children.
The basics are to keep smiling in a friendly way, to engage
in reassuring, distracting conversation, and to touch with great
gentleness, keeping the hands in gliding contact with the skin.
That sounds perfectly straightforward with a child, but with an
adult of the opposite sex might it then have the overtones of a
caress? (Fig. 5.1).

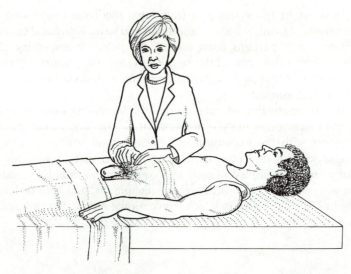

Fig 5.1 The intimacy of clinical touching needs to be 'professionalized'

Anyone who has taught abdominal palpation in pregnancy to medical students will know that they have considerable difficulty in maintaining visual contact with the patient's face, still less in smiling while palpation is in progress. The intimacy of palpation is enough to handle, without the further intimacy of eye-to-eye smiling contact. So the student tends to frown down at his own fingertips (Fig. 5.2) or to gaze with a remote look of intense concentration towards a corner of the ceiling! Meanwhile, the opportunity for the student to convey comfort and reassurance by touch is neglected.

In any case, few patients are likely to relax their abdominal or other musculature unless they can immediately convey discomfort to the doctor by a change of facial expression. It is not enough to instruct 'Tell me if this is sore' or 'Tell me if I am hurting you'. Most patients do not want to make a fuss or a noise during their examination, still less to deter the doctor from finding out what is wrong. So there is nothing for them to do but tense up their muscles protectively and try to be brave. In consequence, the clinical information that can be obtained through palpation is correspondingly reduced. A considerate and sensitive doctor

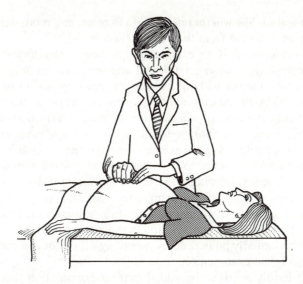

Fig 5.2 Abdominal palpation in pregnancy. The student, feeling awkward, avoids eye-to-eye contact

should therefore avoid touching any part of the patient's body, and possible eliciting tenderness or pain, unless he is keeping the patient's facial expression under observation throughout.

GENTLENESS

Just as the verbal interaction between doctor and patient is a two-way process, information is always conveyed in both directions by the way the doctor touches the patient. Many patients are apprehensive at the prospect of discomfort during physical examination, at the thought that rectal or vaginal examinations may be required, and possibly venepuncture or other painful procedures, perhaps an operation. The doctor's touch, even during a simple initial procedure such as taking the blood pressure, begins to convey a message, which will be one of reassurance only if gentleness is the unvarying rule. Similarly, the considerate gentleness and 'comfort' of the doctor during abdominal examination will reassure a woman who requires vaginal examination that it should not be the ordeal she feared. She will therefore begin to relax, and more information can be obtained from the examination.

Furthermore, if, as examination proceeds, the doctor succeeds in completing the vaginal digital and speculum examination in a sensitive manner without causing any embarrassment or physical discomfort, the *educational* consequences may be far-reaching. For instance, the woman will then not hesitate to return for a regular cervical smear; she will be less likely to book late in pregnancy for fear of a booking vaginal examination; she may feel more confident about seeking contraceptive advice or being fitted with an IUCD; she will be less reluctant to return to the doctor if she subsequently develops gynaecological symptoms. But that may be only the beginning, for the woman may mention how easy the examination was to her female relatives, and perhaps her neighbours. They too can be similarly influenced by spreading echoes of the 'message' of the original examination.

It hardly needs to be added that an examination that conveys feelings of embarrassment or pain will disseminate the opposite sort of message with no less widespread an effect. I have used here the example of vaginal examination, with which I am particularly familiar, but other examples abound. A painful endoscopy, or a botched venepuncture for example, inconsiderately handled in the out-patient clinic, may deter a patient from accepting further treatment as an in-patient. All forms of examination–contact convey indirect educational messages, which can influence whether patients continue to seek help and advice with their health problems.

If gentleness has so much to commend it, facilitating examination and helping to secure the patient's confidence and co-operation, present and future, why should any doctor be heavy handed? In some instances, it may result from lack of physical skill, but in others it can be a manifestation of the doctor's limited comfort and professional assurance, a way of ridding the physical intimacy of touching of any sexual overtones by making it a little uncomfortable, to be on the safe side! The doctor's dis-ease is further expressed by his frown and his 'Tell me if this *hurts*'. One might say, then, that the patient's comfort in a physical sense grows on the doctor's 'comfort' in an affective sense.

If the doctor learns to be truly comfortable with the intimacy of touching in his professional work, then genital examination can be

used both for physical assessment and to help give patients with
sexual dysfunction a new comfort and self-confidence in their own
bodies, which can be an important element in therapy.

In conclusion, it needs to be emphasized that some touch
contacts are wholly negative in the message they convey. For
example, a brief pat on the head or shoulder of a disabled person
in a wheel chair is bound to be perceived as patronizing, reducing
them to the status of a dependent child.

Caring communication skills

The manner in which a doctor communicates with a patient is influenced considerably by the extent to which he feels the need to remain detached from, or is prepared to become involved with, patients' problems and concerns generally, and with their feelings in particular. The extent of the professional 'distance' thus established is readily recognized by the patient. This in turn determines his perception of the doctor's role—of how much involvement he can expect the doctor to show. Some of the ploys which doctors may adopt to maintain greater distance are described on p. 76.

CURING AND CARING

Because of the contrast between detachment and involvement, it is easy to generate a misleading antithesis between curing and caring. Curing is portrayed in this rather stereotyped view as a detached activity on the doctor's part, in which the patient is essentially passive. Caring is taken to imply involvement, a holistic concern with all aspects of the patient's situation. And so a contrast may be drawn between the interventions and technologies of acute medicine associated with episodic illness, and the less dramatic but sustained efforts often required in longer-term care, rehabilitation, etc. The first symbolizes cure; the latter, care.

The idea that such a dichotomy is inherent in the actual practice of medicine has to be challenged. It is quite untrue of family medicine, and even in the subdivided world of hospital medicine a great deal of acute illness presents in the elderly, for instance, and cannot be dissociated from patients' longer-term health problems. It is certainly also a false assumption that the doctor who does relatively more curing (or likes to believe he does!) has less need to be caring, i.e. that quite different attitudes and affective skills are called for in the two situations. Affective aspects of illness are no less evident and important in (say) the intensive-care area than they are in the long-stay geriatric unit.

CARING SKILLS

Curing is fairly easy to define (even if sometimes difficult to achieve), but what does 'caring' mean? The word can be used in different senses in different settings, but in the present context a doctor who cares is not some sort of 'do-gooder', technically rather inept, but always compulsively eager to immerse himself in his patient's emotional problems. He is someone who has trained himself to develop and utilize, in his relationships with patients, certain professional skills. These enable him to handle affective issues and reactions with no less professional competence than he brings to physical or technical problems. The word C-A-R-E provides a simple mnemonic to list important communication skills that the student should strive to develop:

COMFORT

ACCEPTANCE

RESPONSIVENESS

EMPATHY

Each of these skills merits detailed description.

Comfort

This is the ability to deal with emotive topics, matters that may be generally regarded as embarrassing or painful, of which death and sexuality are examples, without becoming uncomfortable. This skill quickly communicates comfort, once the patient has recognized that the doctor is not embarrassed by the topic or situation. Consequently, the patient is not inhibited from talking about what might otherwise have been a subject to avoid, although one central to his problems.

Comfort can apply to situations and circumstances as well as to topics of discussion—to disfigurement, to nudity, to incontinence, to things from which otherwise we might wish to turn away. It is by no means an all-or-nothing skill. Many doctors are comfortable with one topic or situation, but not with another. As we shall see (p. 87), doctors may be particularly uncomfortable when dealing with a problem that mirrors an unresolved conflict or dilemma of their own.

The following examples illustrate absence of comfort with a range of topics that can crop up in everyday practice.

EXAMPLE 1

Doctor	'This is the third time you have asked for a cancer smear in two years, Mrs Anderson. Are you afraid that you have cancer?'
Patient	'Well, um, . . ., yes. I suppose it's the things people say.'
Doctor	'What do they say?'
Patient	'Well, my next door neighbour told me that having intercourse during your period causes cancer and we sometimes do it. But that's quite normal, isn't it, doctor?'
Doctor	(Speaking rather slowly and pompously) 'Well, of course you mustn't listen to things people say. Your doctor is the best person to ask for advice.'
Patient	'Yes, but it is normal, isn't it? I sometimes feel a lot more like sex at my period times.'
Doctor	'Well . . . of course . . . not everybody feels the same about these things. Now I'm going to take a smear when nurse comes back and you won't need another one for four years. Just go behind the screen and take off your . . . er . . . get ready for me to examine you.'

EXAMPLE 2

Consultant	'Now, Mrs MacLeod, we have examined you from top to toe and I am pleased to be able to tell you that I can find no sign of any physical disease, and all the tests have come back negative. I think you need to start getting out and about more. You have a daughter, born . . . let's see . . . she must

	be 16 now. You and she could go out together for company.'
Patient	'Doctor . . . my daughter is dead! Elaine started sniffing glue when she was just 13 and last year it killed her.'
Consultant	'Oh! I'm terribly sorry!' (Looks away) 'How dreadful!' (Pauses and hesitates) 'Look, Mrs MacLeod I'm going to prescribe for you a new and very effective antidepressant drug. I'm sure this will help you get back to normal again.'

EXAMPLE 3

Consultant	(To a young soldier who is recovering from disfiguring burns of the face and hands) 'Now, Robert. I think we'll be able to get most of those bandages off tomorrow for good!'
Young Soldier	'I'm not sure I'd not be better off with them on. I've watched the nurses' eyes when they're doing my dressings! Doctor, do you think anyone will ever be able to bear the sight of me?'
Consultant	(Immediately turning away and addressing his remarks to the group at the foot of the bed in a loud pontifical voice) 'Sister, it sounds as if Robert's morale is a bit low today. You'll have to get his visitors to cheer him up.'
Young Soldier	(To the now retreating figure of the consultant) 'The only visitor I want to see is Angela, but she's not been near the place for more than a fortnight! I don't think she wants me anymore!'

EXAMPLE 4

Doctor	'Now tell me about your family, Mrs Bishop. You have a family?'
Patient	'Yes, I have three sons. They are 24, 17, and 16 years old now.'
Doctor	'Are they all in good health?'
Patient	'Yes.'
Doctor	'You must be proud of them! Are you a granny yet?'
Patient	'No. My eldest son will never marry, I don't

suppose. You see, doctor, he's . . . er . . . a homosexual.'

Doctor
'Oh!' I *am* sorry! I'm sorry I asked! I didn't mean to embarrass you. The other two are normal, I suppose?'

EXAMPLE 5

Consultant
(On ward round, from the foot of the bed) 'Good morning, Mr Grimes. And how are we today?' (Note the impersonal patronizing 'we')

Patient
(Who looks very ill and has obviously lost a lot of weight) 'I'm not feeling so good today. I keep being sick. Doctor . . . can I have a word with you?'

Consultant
'Why, certainly! What can we do for you?' (Note the distant 'we' again)

Patient
'Doctor, tell me straight. Is it serious? I want to know. Have I got much of a chance?'

Consultant
(With a rather empty smile) 'Well, . . . er . . . we're not . . . er . . . exactly sure just at the minute how . . . er . . . active this little growth in your stomach is. But we've got some more tests and ideas up our sleeves, you know. So keep your chin up, Mr Grimes.'

EXAMPLE 6

Patient
'Doctor, my nerves have just gone to pieces since I lost my husband last year. I'm so lonely. It was so sudden. I still can't accept it. He was only 38! Now I'm terribly worried about myself.'

Doctor
'What are you worrying about?'

Patient
'Oh, just my health and . . . well . . . doctor, I must tell you. Since I lost my husband I have started masturbating . . . er . . . occasionally. Sometimes I feel very dirty, and sometimes it really helps. (Remains silent for a moment with her head lowered) Do you think I'm dreadful?'

Doctor
'Oh, come on now, Mrs Black! You're letting your nerves get the better of you. (Pauses) You'll have to pull yourself together. I'm . . . er . . . I'm going

to give you some tablets to help calm you down a bit. You must get them from the chemist right away and start taking them three times a day after meals. Have you got that clear now, three times a day after meals?'

In each of the above examples, the doctor has revealed his discomfort with a topic implicated in his patient's problem. In consequence, the patient is unlikely to be willing to mention that topic again, either with the same doctor, or possibly even with other doctors.

Absence of comfort can sometimes be revealed in a subtle way, just by the choice of words. The use of a stilted euphemism can immediately betray the doctor's dis-ease. For example, the doctor, trying to ask a patient about possible sexual abuse as a child might enquire 'Did you ever receive any . . . er . . . shall we say unwelcome attentions . . . when you were younger, that is?', or wishing to enquire about possible extramarital sexual contact might ask 'Have you ever been . . . er . . . tempted from the straight and narrow, so to speak?', or seeking evidence of alcohol abuse could ask 'Do you . . . shall we say . . . over-indulge?' Or suppose the doctor initiates enquiries about sexual function in a similarly hesitant and stilted way with phrases such as 'Now, Mrs Black, is everything all right at home? Is the . . . er . . . physical side of your . . . er . . . married life satisfactory?' The patient is bound to sense the doctor's awkwardness and feel inhibited in replying. Nor is the patient likely to be put at ease if the doctor in this situation resorts to the use of sexual slang or false jocularity. Even a phrase such as 'your sex-life' is usually best avoided. It is too familiar, and its use may weaken the sense of formal professional correctness. It is best to choose a simple but direct and explicit form of words: 'Do you and your wife have a good sexual relationship?' 'Are you able to enjoy sexual intercourse without discomfort?', or in the case of an older person 'Are you still able to have sexual intercourse satisfactorily?' These questions are clear and unambiguous. When the doctor maintains eye contact while asking the question, his comfort with, and willingness to talk about, the topic are conveyed.

Comfort can be learned through regular repeated exposure to sensitive topics, in an environment where the learner can share his feelings with others in a peer group. Familiarity need not breed contempt; the doctor can retain his sensibility while shedding his discomfort. The development of comfort is facilitated by the acquisition of relevant vocabulary and phraseology which make it easier to discuss awkward topics.

Acceptance

This refers to the ability to accept the feelings and attitudes the patient brings to the interview, without allowing them to prevent good rapport and communication. Sometimes these are feelings associated with illness that are liable to irritate or anger the doctor, such as irrational fear or mistrust, anger or resentment, undue reticence, inadequacy, or apathy.

The patient may appear over-dependent and feckless, unwilling to assume any responsibility for his own health, but expecting the doctor to produce some instant 'cure' for his ills. At the other end of the spectrum, he may be a critical intellectual, untrusting and always ready to propose some alternative to the doctor's suggestions; or he may be endlessly demanding and manipulative. These attitudes may irritate the doctor beyond endurance. Again, he may sometimes resent strongly the time spent on certain patient's problems, which appear largely self-imposed: the fruits of an unhealthy lifestyle which the patient is reluctant to change, such as obesity in the gourmand or chronic dyspepsia due to alcohol abuse, repeated pelvic infection associated with promiscuity, or bronchitis in a heavy smoker. In other instances the doctor may feel alienated before a word is spoken because of the patient's cultural trappings, whether it be the young 'punk' with shaved head and safety-pin ear-rings, the pretentious dame with lacquered blue rinse and podgy over-gemmed fingers, or the vapid 'New-Ager', decked with 'active' bangle and pendant crystal.

It is therefore essential that the doctor should not be blind to his own cultural, social, and moral prejudices, so that these personal attitudes, which all of us possess in some degree, are not allowed to obstruct the development of rapport and trust. Prejudice apart, the more the doctor learns to recognize and understand his own attitudes and motives in his professional work, the more he will be able to understand and help his patients. Self-awareness is at the heart of professional competence.

Acceptance does not imply that the doctor should not seek in the course of time to change the patient's attitudes, if that seems a necessary part of treatment. It means that the doctor always treats the patient with respect, and endeavours to discover *why* the patient feels or behaves as he does, and equally why he himself may be antagonized by the patient's behaviour. This insight helps to prevent the doctor from reacting in a way that hinders understanding and blocks communication between the patient and himself.

The patient's personal and family history often sheds light on his attitudes in the present illness. For example, a period spent in hospital as a small child, for (say) tonsillectomy, may leave behind a lifelong fear of hospitals, sometimes deserving the term 'hospital phobia'. Even visits during childhood to a dying close relative in hospital may have a similar effect. A relative's or friend's death from cancer can leave a legacy of obsessive fear. Sometimes the patient gains insight and reassurance when the significance of past experiences are explained. The patient may be well aware of the irrational or unacceptable nature of his feelings, but unable to control them. The fact that he senses the doctor is accepting him as he is can greatly facilitate their relationship.

Again, it is common for the mother of young children who is unsupported through single-parenthood, divorce, separation, or widowhood to be beset by anxiety about her own health, especially when she is the family's sole breadwinner. Her awareness of the children's dependence on her well-being may constantly cloud her thoughts with irrational fear, and she may appear indifferent to reassurance.

Sometimes patients' previous experiences with doctors may have generated deep distrust. At worst, a patient may initially describe his problems in terms which are more or less a catalogue of criticisms or accusations against his previous medical attendants. If a doctor senses such suspicion or hostility early in the interview— if the patient shows a questioning, critical or resentful attitude from the outset—it is wise to go over the management of previous illnesses at the earliest opportunity in an open way, to see if the origin of the patient's mistrust can be identified, and perhaps 'defused'.

However assiduously a doctor endeavours to demonstrate acceptance during interaction with patients, from time to time occasional individuals seem impossibly difficult. One may show mistrust and aggression; another is persistently unco-operative and demanding, manipulative or obstructive.

Faced with such situations, it may be next to impossible in the course of a single consultation to achieve rapport, or even to take first steps towards a constructive relationship. Because of the antipathy aroused, and because the doctor may feel unsure how he can make any progress, he may be sorely tempted to bring the interview to an end in a deliberately negative way, conveying the implicit message that he does not wish to see the patient again—ever!

'I'm afraid then there's little or nothing I can do for you—nothing that hasn't been tried before without any apparent benefit.'

'Well, if that's how you feel, you'd really better get another opinion from someone you perhaps **will** have confidence in. I'm wasting my time trying to help you.'

Breaking off in this way will make acceptance well nigh impossible in the future. It should not be done impulsively, therefore, but only if the doctor is morally certain that he cannot help the patient in any way. If he is unsure at the end of a single interview whether an effective relationship can be established, it is better to buy time for another look at the situation. He might, for example, take a blood test or two, asking the patient to return when the results are available; or he might put the patient's sincerity to the test by seeking his active co-operation, asking him to keep a diary of his symptom pattern, or recommending some change in habits and lifestyle before seeing him again.

As doctors become aware of the importance of acceptance, they learn not to use such trite and uncomprehending remarks as 'You are going to be fine, cheer up!', 'Don't look so worried, there is *nothing* to worry about!', 'This examination will not bother you *at all*', or 'Now, you'll just have to pull yourself together!'

Acceptance is promoted by learning more about the lifestyles and cultures of others, and seeking to understand the factors which shape people's attitudes and values, including the doctor's own. *Tout comprendre, c'est tout pardonner!* Although there may well remain limits to a doctor's ability to demonstrate acceptance, he should at least be aware of those limits, and ready to acknowledge them.

Responsiveness

This is the skill of reacting to indirect or incomplete 'messages' that are put out by the patient during an interview. The essential element of the skill is not just in making the responses, but in the sensitive alertness that first recognizes the clue or cue, an indication that here is something about which more needs to be said, some affective topic that the patient might be reluctant to bring into the open without prompting, or feels unsure whether it is appropriate to discuss. The clue might be an inflection of the voice, a hesitation, a gesture or some other signal in body language, or a more overt but oblique reference to a problem.

As was described in Chapter 3, it is often best to respond to such clues *at the time*, and therefore to diverge from the previous line of enquiry. Sometimes, however, it is wiser not to divert from what the patient is in the middle of saying, but to come back later to the matter that has only barely been hinted at.

Consider, as simple examples, the possible variety of replies to a common question such as 'And is your husband in good health?':

(i) *Patient*   'Oh! you will have to ask *him* about that!', hinting that 'He and I don't share much communication about personal things', or even meaning 'He is the sort of man who would be very angry if he thought I was talking to you about his health behind his back.'
The doctor might respond with something like 'Why? Does he not talk much about himself?'

(ii) *Patient*   'Oh, there is never anything wrong with *him*', hinting 'And that's why *I* get very little sympathy!'
The doctor might respond 'Do you think he understands how *you* feel then?'

(iii) *Patient*   (Warmly) 'He has never had a day's illness in his life, I look after him so well!', indicating that 'We have a close and secure relationship.'

(iv) *Patient*   'Well' (patient pauses and speaks very quietly) 'actually . . .' (patient suddenly appears about to be overcome by feeling) 'I would rather not talk about that now.'

The doctor, responding immediately, might remain silent for a few moments, then leaning forward ask quietly 'Why, is it a big worry for you? Perhaps you could tell me *something* about it?'

Similarly, consider the varied replies one might hear to the question 'And have you always up to now enjoyed good health?':

(i) *Patient* 'Well . . . (long pause) . . . generally, I suppose . . . not too bad. I've never had anything serious *before*.'

The doctor might respond 'And are you thinking it might be serious *now*?'

(ii) *Patient* 'Oh, I couldn't say that! People at work are *always* telling me I don't look well.'

The doctor might respond 'And does that upset you? Does it get you down?'

(iii) *Patient* 'Yes. I've always been fit as a flea. Never had a day's illness in my life . . . up till *now*.'

The doctor might respond 'So what are you thinking about having to go into hospital now?'

(iv) *Patient* 'Well. I don't suppose I've ever had what *you* would call an illness. But I don't *ever* feel well. I think I've been suffering from "nerves" for years . . . ever since I was a girl at school.'

The doctor might respond 'And what do you think happened then to start it off?' or 'Do you feel other people don't understand how unwell you feel?'

Here is another example, illustrating how the doctor's responsiveness can influence the direction of an interview.

Doctor 'You have had this discharge for some time?'
Patient 'Two years now, ever since the baby came.'
Doctor 'Does it make you feel itchy?'
Patient 'Sometimes.'
Doctor 'Does it have an unpleasant odour?'
Patient 'Yes, it does.' (Looks away, dropping her voice)
Doctor (Quickly) 'What colour is it?'

Patient 'Well, it's difficult to describe, darkish I suppose.'
Doctor 'But is it white or yellow or green or brown?'
Patient 'It could be any of those colours at different times.'
Doctor (Impatiently) 'You can't tell me what colour it is, then?'

Let us see how this interview might have gone with an appropriate response from the doctor.

Doctor 'Does it have an unpleasant odour?'
Patient 'Yes, it does.' (Looks away, dropping her voice)
Doctor (Responding to the patient's subdued reply) 'You feel self-conscious about it? Do you think other people would be aware of it?'
Patient 'Well . . . Yes . . . my husband certainly. When it was bad last year, he made remarks about it. I just avoid letting him come near me now.'
Doctor 'And has anyone, apart from your husband, said anything?'
Patient 'Well, not actually. But I'm always afraid that other people notice. I don't go out much socially nowadays. I never feel comfortable in company.'

Responsiveness is a skill which depends first and foremost on active observant listening. The character and detail of the doctor's responses cannot, of course, be prescribed. The effectiveness of the responses depends on recognizing that the patient is saying, or trying to say, something important; and then attempting to convey through the response the doctor's readiness to listen further, and his concern and understanding.

Empathy

Empathic remarks are a commonplace of everyday friendly conversation wherever people are communicating in a warm cordial way: 'You must have felt on top of the world!' 'How awful!' 'I bet you were mad with him!' 'Didn't you want to scream?' 'What a shame' 'Great!' 'Marvellous!'

These varied responses all convey a similar message: 'I know how you feel or felt. I could feel much the same in the same situation, and so I view your feelings, happy, sad, angry, confused or whatever, as appropriate. I endorse them.' Empathic responses do *not* signify that the speaker is experiencing the same feelings. But he is indicating that he shares them to the extent that he recognizes and understands them, and acknowledging that he would probably, if placed in similar circumstances, have similar feelings.

Empathy is, then, a limited but positive response to the feelings experienced by another person, whether these feelings are expressed openly or not. It is not an indifferent aloofness or an open rejection of the other person's feelings, nor is it a sympathetic joining in the feelings. It signifies a middle way which nevertheless expresses understanding and promotes openness and warmth between the speakers.

However, the doctor must keep in mind that each patient's feelings are experienced as something very personal to that individual. It is quite unhelpful, therefore, to declare directly 'I *know* just how you feel!' The personal quality of someones else's distress (or elation) has to be 'shared' in a more oblique and less presumptuous way. In the occasional instance when a doctor has indeed personally been through a similar experience to the patient, however, he may by revealing this be able to create a basis for special mutual understanding.

After Don Homrich married Terri Nelson (another heart-transplant survivor) in 1988, he said 'We've both been through the same thing so we know what it's like. When some people say "I know how you feel", I hate that! When *she* says she knows how I feel, she really does!'

These telling remarks illustrate that a patient experiencing distress can often best, and sometimes only receive support from someone who has had the same experience. Hence the special value of helping groups such as Cruse (for widows), the Mastectomy Association, and many others for particular disorders. Even those with relatively rare disorders can make contact with other similarly affected families through the Contact with Families group. In such groups, a true sharing of feelings (which is something closer and deeper than empathy) is possible.

The use of empathy does not necessarily depend upon the patient openly expressing his feelings. The most empathic remarks can be made when a doctor is able, from experience or intuition, to sense the patient's feelings correctly even before he mentions them, and so convey his own understanding of the situation. Sometimes also he can try to help the patient to put difficult feelings into words. Even if the doctor guesses wrongly about the feeling, it will not be unhelpful, so long as his tentative assumption is expressed in a warm, friendly way, possibly as a question. (See also p. 167).

'And did this attack of pain in your chest make you feel afraid— really afraid?'

'I guess you must have felt quite anxious when you saw the blood in your urine?'

'Was your wife's behaviour making you feel more and more resentful—and even jealous?'

Here are one or two examples of the way in which an empathic remark can influence the character of an interview.

Doctor 'How long have you been married?'
Patient 'Six years, doctor.'
Doctor And is this your first pregnancy?'
Patient 'Oh no, doctor! I have had a miscarriage.'
Doctor When was that?'
Patient 'In April 1976.'
Doctor How far on were you?'
Patient 'Oh, only 10 weeks.'
Doctor Did you have the womb scraped out afterwards?'
Patient 'Yes, I had to have a D&C.'
Doctor Which hospital was that?'
Patient 'I was staying in Birmingham at the time. I can't remember the name of the hospital.'
Doctor Try to remember it. You see, it's quite important that I write to get all the particulars. Can you give me *any* lead where it was? What was the doctor's name?'

The patient now feels inadequate, unable to help the doctor in what he obviously feels are important enquiries. But beyond that, the patient has had no opportunity to convey to the doctor how she feels about her first pregnancy. He has appeared to be concerned only with the physical events of the miscarriage, and oblivious to her reactions to those events, which she has had no opportunity to express.

Now let us pick up that interview again part way through, and see the difference when an empathic response is made by the doctor.

Doctor 'How far on were you?'

Patient   'Oh, only 10 weeks.'
Doctor   'Had you been trying for a pregnancy for long?'
Patient   'Yes, for about three years.'
Doctor   *'That must have been a terrible disappointment for you!'*
Patient   'Yes, it was like the end of the world! My husband was so
            disappointed too. I felt miserable for months afterwards.
            I suppose that's why I'm so worried this time. Now I
            daren't let myself believe that I'm going to have a baby.

Here is another simple example of how the introduction of an
empathic remark might open up the conversation.

Doctor   'Are your parents both alive?'
Patient   'No, my mother died in 1968.'
Doctor   What was the matter with her?'
Patient   'I think it was cancer, doctor.'
Doctor   In what part of the body?'
Patient   'I am not sure.'
Doctor   'Did she have an operation? Was it in this hospital? Can
            you tell me anything about it?'

Now see the difference an empathic response brings.

Doctor   'Are your parents both alive?'
Patient   'No, my mother died in 1968.'
Doctor   (Pausing) *'You were only 12 then!'*
Patient   'Yes, it really was the last of my childhood. I had to
            help my father look after her when she came home from
            hospital. She had cancer, you know. Actually, I often
            think about her. I keep hoping the same thing never
            happens to me.'

Empathy, we see, provides an appropriate controlled, professional
response to the patient's affective reaction to illness. It not only
assures the patient that his doctor understands how he feels but
most importantly it *protects* the doctor, delimiting the extent of his
affective involvement with the patient's problem.

The student needs to appreciate clearly the limits implied in
responding with empathy. Those involved in the task of caring *have*
to maintain an appropriate professional distance. When doctors are
criticized for their professional aloofness, it is often asserted that
they ought to display more humanity. Indeed, humanity in dealing

with patients is a declared learning goal of the curriculum in some medical schools. But the natural spontaneous human reaction to the distress of another person is sympathy—a true sharing of painful emotion (literally, 'suffering together'). This is a burden that becomes unsupportable when it is constantly borne. It is not surprising, therefore, that the phenomenon of 'burn out' [37] is liable gradually to overwhelm those whose commitment to the business of caring is too long and too deeply sustained. Some may feel drawn to be involved in this way because of circumstances in their own upbringing. They may not have fully recognized the wise limits that need to be set to their emotional involvement, or their need for continuing peer support.

Besides, an outpouring of sympathy by the doctor, sharing in the patient's distress, could well inhibit the patient from expressing the true depths of his feelings, out of a wish to spare the doctor.

The ability to use empathy effectively as a professional skill to facilitate communication depends on acquiring, through listening and reading, and sometimes through personal or family experiences of illness, a more complete understanding of how patients are likely to feel in particular situations. Young doctors have not all faced an operation for the removal of a leg or a breast or a uterus; had a stroke; experienced an unexpected bereavement or a miscarriage; had a doubtful cervical smear; become diabetic; discovered they carry a familial risk of genetic disease; been told that they have high blood pressure, rheumatoid arthritis, Parkinson's disease, or cancer. But though one may know almost all there is to know about a disease, one can still learn more about how it feels to actually experience it [38]. In this regard, various leaflets and booklets produced by patient associations and similar helping groups provide a great deal of first-hand information [39,40].

A series of Personal Papers published in the *Lancet* (1967–75), describing doctors' personal experiences of serious illness, provide another invaluable source of insight. Many of these doctor-patients recalled with feeling the distress they had experienced because of inadequate communication, especially of an affective kind, between their attendants and themselves. Their concerns as patients were often not recognized or were ignored, their anxieties went unrelieved, and they commonly felt in the dark, despite their medical knowledge. Although they might have had the privilege of carefully choosing their medical attendant, they often ended up thinking that the person they had chosen did not really understand how they felt.

These writings apart, each doctor's own clinical work should provide him with an ever-expanding fund of knowledge about how people feel when they experience ill health. So long as a doctor has an ear to listen, and so long as he does not inhibit the expression of affect, he can continually add to his capacity for empathic responsiveness.

The experience which is, perhaps, the most difficult to share empathically is the approach of death. This is not only because it is an experience which provides no opportunity for retrospective description, but also because of the resistance to putting oneself in the dying patient's shoes.

These four behavioural skills—comfort, acceptance, responsiveness, and empathy—help to equip the doctor to handle the affective dimensions of patients' problems with no less competence than those of a technical nature. The first two, comfort and acceptance, are skills that help the professional to control expression on his part of negative and often disruptive affective responses.

The latter two skills, responsiveness and empathy, are concerned with the doctor's positive professional responses to affect, by which he recognizes and elucidates feelings that the patient may have only hinted at. He learns to react not with indifference or aloofness, nor with effusive unproductive sympathy, but with a human response that is professionally caring and helpful to the patient but which does not subject himself to an intolerable burden of emotional stress.

7 Obstacles to communication

The time available for an interview varies from doctor to doctor, and from day to day. The conduct of the interview is bound to be influenced by this constraint, but the doctor must not let the pressure of time cramp his interviewing style in a way that inhibits open communication. In contemporary hospital practice, more rapid turnover in the wards, the growth of high-technology, high-dependency care, and expanding day-case care have all progressively increased the pressures on staff. Doctors and nurses alike are often short of time, have to watch over monitors as well as patients, and may be, at times, short of sleep. The quest for cost-efficiency itself involves many obstacles to communication.

In general practice [41–44] and in some busy hospital clinics, the average time available per patient may be only 5–10 minutes, although a little more time is often allocated to 'new' patients. In a less pressured general medical clinic, 30 minutes or more might be available, and most psychiatrists prefer to spend a full hour with a new patient. In each of these settings, therefore, a different pace and style of interviewing needs to be adopted. In the private health-care system of the United States, the average consultation time is about 18 minutes.

Obviously, the shape of an interview depends largely on whether it is a first consultation or a renewal of contact in the course of continuing care. For instance, in many general practice consultations, the doctor already knows much that he has learnt about the patient in previous contacts.

I doubt whether it is necessary, or indeed helpful in a first interview, to declare at the beginning how much time is available. Such a statement might appear as an attempt to curtail communication, rather than to facilitate it. However, it may be a useful thing to do at a subsequent interview. Sometimes one has to decide whether to attempt to complete an interview there and then, or to agree and plan with the patient a second instalment, when more time may be available.

When a further interview is anticipated, the doctor has greater freedom to plan the stages of the consultation. He may decide, for example, not to conduct a full physical examination during the first visit; he may deliberately defer exploration of the patient's close personal relationships until a second or even a third interview; he may leave the exposition (p. 121) until a subsequent appointment. In these circumstances the patient should always be given an explanation of how and why the stages of the whole consultation are to proceed.

The doctor should try to appear unhurried and ready to listen, even when time is limited. Any evidence that he is short of time is likely to be spotted by the patient, who will then be less willing to open up. If the patient enters the room to find the doctor hurriedly completing case notes or pathology forms, or dashing through a phone call, or if the doctor hustles the nurse or, remaining standing, jumps straight to the presenting complaint, the interview will be constricted by a sense of haste. Richard Asher [20] put it well: 'To give a patient the impression you could spare him an hour, and yet make him satisfied within five minutes, is an invaluable gift, and of much more use than spending half an hour with him, during every minute of which he is made to feel he is encroaching on your time!'

But when time *is* at a premium, the consultation *has* to be streamlined to match the time available. In this situation, it is even more important that patients should feel they have enough time to describe their problems. Wilkinson [45] reported and compared two series of 100 patients each in general practice and a consultant clinic. Every patient was afforded time to speak without interruption about his complaint(s). Table 7.1 shows for how long the patients spoke.

It can be seen that 98 per cent of patients in general practice and 70 per cent in hospital consultations took less than 2 minutes to describe their complaint. Even in hospital consultations, only one patient in five needed 4 minutes or more.

Using selective questions, the skill and experience of the practitioner pays dividends, through his ability to formulate a logical

Table 7.1 Percentage distribution of time needed to describe initial complaint. (From Wilkinson [45].)

	<60'	60'–120'	2–3 min	≥4 min	Mean time
General practice	75	23	1	1	43s
Consultation	42	28	11	19	1 min 40s

sequence of enquiries that leads via the least number of diagnostic steps towards a presumptive diagnosis. But the learner needs to remind himself repeatedly that medical diagnosis is in very many instances a statement of probability, rather than the elucidation of an absolute truth. One could spend half a lifetime looking for certainty, but medical decisions are almost always constrained by time.

On occasion, an over-talkative patient will begin to take up an inordinate amount of time, embarking on a sequence of irrelevant items of gossip or introspective trivia. The patient may be a lonely character, for whom a visit to the doctor can provide a wonderful conversational outlet full of reminiscence, or he may be a born talker who turns every encounter into a self-centred monologue. The doctor, listening impatiently, may detect features of obsession or anxiety, manipulative fiction, or the stale smell of alcohol.

In each such encounter, the doctor has to draw his own lines, in a responsible way, between therapeutic listening and unproductive time-wasting. If he feels that the patient's rambling loquacity is seriously wasting his time, he should attempt to maintain control of the dialogue without losing the patient's confidence. It may sometimes be appropriate to say directly something like 'Now, Mrs Robertson, I'm very pressed for time today. Just try to answer my questions, and leave it at that.' If the doctor feels he needs to be more subtle, he can ask the patient to undress partially, which tends to inhibit the patient. More simply, he can bring out his stethoscope and make a show of auscultating the chest, or even put a thermometer in the patient's mouth! Most patients are less inclined to chatter if there is also a nurse present, so it may help to recall the nurse if she has left the room.

THE PROBLEMS OF PAIN, SUFFERING, AND DEATH

As already discussed, doctors need some protective insulation from the emotional distress that can be generated by the pain, suffering, death, and bereavement encountered in the course of clinical work. They therefore need to develop an understanding of how these influences, and that of death in particular, affect communication between doctor and patient [46].

Although death is the one certainty in each of our futures, the common lot of all humanity, it is something which people are reluctant to contemplate or to discuss. Since, during the present century, death in childhood or in youth has become a rarity and life expectation has extended, people usually prefer to keep dying out of mind. The majority, for example, never get round to writing a will.

To detach themselves from the painful feelings associated with serious illness and death, doctors may elect, almost unconsciously, to avoid eliciting from their patients expression of *any* distressing feelings, and may be inclined, therefore, to adopt a rather distant and impersonal attitude in clinical work generally. Maguire [47] described the following ploys which doctors may use to distance themselves from their patients' feelings:

• restricting the focus of discussion to non-emotive topics;

• diverting the focus of discussion away from possibly emotive topics;

• playing down the feelings as 'normal';

• blanketing the patient with over-reassurance;

• using leading questions; pre-empting the replies;

• jollying the patient along, with platitudes and clichés.

Specifically, they can often find the utmost difficulty in speaking honestly with the patient whose illness is likely to be mortal. In many instances they may have recourse to evasion, silence, half-truths, or even deliberate deception. The misleading assumptions that underlie this behaviour run as follows. People do not want to die, therefore they do not want to know that they are dying. They could not tolerate being told that they are dying, nor do they recognize that they are dying. If the patient is fobbed off with glib reassurance or falsities, he will soon realize that the doctor feels he cannot share the truth with him. This creates a sense of isolation and lack of trust. The experience is made more lonely since there is no one who can empathize and say 'That's just how I felt when I was dying.'

The consequence of this unwillingness to acknowledge the moment of truth that mortal illness almost inevitably brings are usually disastrous for the doctor–patient relationship. Confidence, trust, and rapport are likely to melt away, and cannot subsequently be restored. The patient's close relatives may be taken aside and given a true account of the patient's condition, but made accomplices in the attempt to deceive. When they in turn later become patients, they already know how the pretence is staged. In this way a doctor can in large measure destroy his ability to reassure those patients whose illness is not in fact serious, for his word is no longer regarded as trustworthy.

But nothing is gained when evasive deception is merely replaced by a routine policy of blunt frankness. Some patients need time—a period of adjustment—to recognize and acknowledge that their illness is mortal. Having adopted denial as protection against their worst fears, they may be overwhelmed by despair or anger if, in the hurried environment of a busy clinic or ward, they are confronted with a bald pronouncement [48].

If doctors are to equip themselves to bring help and support to patients who face terminal illness, one prerequisite is greater understanding of the emotions associated with the prospect of death. Much of this knowledge derives from studies carried out in the hospice movement. Hinton [49] and Kubler-Ross [50] described five phases of emotional reaction that the patient who faces dying is likely to experience. Between the initial feelings of denial or disbelief and the eventual acceptance of what will be, the patient may pass through phases of anger and resentment, bargaining, and depression. A clearer understanding of this range of feelings is the basis on which empathic support rests.

Those who are mortally ill or suffering in other ways may search within themselves for an answer to the question 'Why me?' In some instances, feelings of guilt or self-blame can arise. The illness may be seen as a form of requital for past wrongdoing—the pay-off, the karma of oriental religion. These feelings can sometimes make acceptance of the situation easier for the patient.

Bereavement

In addition to a greater understanding of the varied emotions which may be felt by patients who are dying, we now recognize more clearly the need for the bereaved to acknowledge and express grief and mourning [51,52,53]. Too often, the conspiracy of silence and aversion that surrounds death encompasses the bereaved family, denying them proper opportunities to express their grief, which may be manifested not just as sadness, but as anger or apathy, denial, questioning, or resignment. The reactions to bereavement and the pattern of mourning vary a great deal in different ethnic communities [54] (see Chapter 20), and in different age groups.

As well as showing sensitive awareness of how individual relatives may wish to express their grief, the professionals concerned need not suppress their own reactions to a patient's death. It can be helpful to tell the family what made their relative special, and how he or she will be missed and remembered by the staff. Above all, there is no place for trite remarks such as 'It's all for the best. She wouldn't ever have been normal, even if she had pulled through', or, in the case of a pregnancy loss

'Still, I'm sure you'll soon be able to try again'.

In my own specialty, obstetrics, it seems particularly difficult to come to terms with death, grief, and mourning. Doctors and midwives alike are geared to expect a successful outcome from pregnancy and childbirth. Still birth is now such a rarity that we are ill prepared to cope with it, whereas miscarriage is so common that the mother's sense of grievous loss is often overlooked or brushed aside [56,57]. After an unsuccessful pregnancy, the grieving mother seems quite out of place in the happy atmosphere of a maternity unit. Her tears may be wrongly seen as an indication to administer a sedative drug. She is likely to be put into a single room, which staff may be reluctant to enter, not knowing what to say or how to comfort her. Opportunities to acknowledge and express her grief are thus denied her.

Guidelines from the Royal College of Obstetricians and Gynaecologists and from the Still birth and Neonatal Death Association set out the points of importance. Following still birth, it may greatly help the parents to come to terms with their loss if they are offered the opportunity to see and touch their infant, even in instances where there is some congenital abnormality. It can also be helpful if the stillborn infant is photographed, so that parents who subsequently wish for some record of their child can be given the print [55].

A feeling of bereavement and a need to grieve can follow losses other than death [58]. These include:

- loss or breakdown of a close relationship;
- loss of a part of the body (a limb, a breast) or of a faculty;
- loss of employment, or job status;
- loss of personal treasured possessions.

These brief references to the distressing feelings aroused by death and bereavement provide a very incomplete account of this neglected topic, which is so important in its influence upon the practice of medicine. If the doctor is unable to contemplate death and dying with equanimity, he may erect for his own defence yet another emotional curtain that is likely to isolate him in a wider way from the affective aspects of illness.

Death and suffering remain tragic enigmas of the human condition. But doctors have a special need to come to terms with these emotive experiences and not to allow their professional caring role to be diminished because they feel uncomfortable when confronted with the prospect of death. Specifically, doctors in training for clinical practice should make it their business to acquire the skills used in the care of the dying and the bereaved. To achieve this they have to overcome resistances within themselves, while at the same time learning more about the physical needs of the dying: about the relief of intractable pain, vomiting, dyspnoea, or other physical distress; about the pattern of emotional reaction during terminal illness; about the most appropriate language to use when facing the insecurity of patients and the anxieties of relatives. It can be helpful for the learner to see the family along with a more experienced doctor or nurse; to discuss beforehand the approach; and to give each other feedback and support afterwards. Black *et al* [59] reviewed the education of medical students on death and dying, and identified the more important learning objectives in this area.

In Chapter 17, Dr Derek Doyle, from his wide experience at St Columba's Hospice, Edinburgh, discusses the special skills of talking with the dying. As skill is developed, it will come to be recognized increasingly that patients can indeed 'die well', and that doctors' and nurses' expertise can be a crucial influence in such a situation.

THE PROBLEM OF SEXUALITY

We have seen earlier the basic requirement that the physical intimacy of clinical examination has to be professionalized, and so rendered safe for both patient and doctor. In effect, this means that clinical contacts have to be dissociated from sexual connotations or feelings which, in other settings, might be evoked by nakedness and intimate touching. In consequence, the patient can feel at ease and secure, and the doctor is not exposed to disturbing or intolerable feelings. A majority of male and a minority of female doctors acknowledge that they do sometimes experience feelings of sexual attraction towards patients. Actual sexual contact, though much less common, usually destroys the professional relationship [60].

This neutralization of sexual feelings and reactions is not something affecting only the doctor. Equally important is the patient's perception of the correctness of the professional relationship, how secure he or she feels. This is influenced by the patient's cultural background. It will not be the same for (say) a former Pakistani villager woman as for a local city-born university graduate.

There is little explicit teaching in medical schools about how to desexualize the nudity and intimate touching encountered in clinical work, and the subject is rarely discussed. Perhaps the topic is thought too sensitive to be aired, and it is hoped that, by not giving the matter any consideration, it will assume less significance, so that clinical work will cease to have a sexual connotation. But doctors and nurses need to be able to discuss these issues openly during their training, without feeling that they might therefore be stigmatized, or ridiculed by their teachers as 'weird'.

Several features of the doctor's style and behaviour help to bring about this desexualization: formal clothing (in hospital, often a white coat); a serious demeanour; formal correctness of address; a detached manner, giving no indication of any affective response to the intimacy of clinical contact. Conventionally, a chaperone is arranged if the doctor and the patient are adults of the opposite sex, and this tradition lives on, not so much because most patients in contemporary times expect it, or indeed feel more at ease when a chaperone is present, but probably because it provides the doctor with legal protection from any accusation of impropriety. The Medical Protection Society advises that 'a chaperone should ideally be present when intimate examinations are performed' [61]. However, a postal questionnaire among 171 male general practitioners showed that only 13 per cent always use a chaperone when examining female patients and 25 per cent never do so [62].

These trappings of professionally 'correct' behaviour may still not provide enough protection for some doctors, who might feel over-conscious of their good name and of the need to avoid the faintest imputation of familiarity; or who may find it genuinely difficult to rid the clinical relationship of all sexual connotation. Such individuals may, perhaps unconsciously, find it necessary to exclude any thought or discussion of the patient's sexuality from the clinical situation. But in a more general way, because of this wish not to be 'too personal', some doctors may therefore find it difficult to discuss the patient's close relationships and feelings *at all*. As a consequence, the patient may be seen in a rather narrow, distorted perspective, which more or less ignores the social context of his ill health. The doctor's lack of insight can, at the worst, produce a situation in which his relationship with the patient is not only desexualized, but virtually dehumanized. It has become 'clinical' in the very *worst* sense of the word (page 9).

If the doctor does not understand the factors influencing his professional behaviour, he may secure for himself a cloak of professional correctness, but only a very limited degree of inward comfort. He may, for example, be at ease when examining certain parts of the body that are within his clinical ambit, but not others that are outside his everyday routines. A physician or surgeon might be perfectly at ease performing a rectal examination, but averse to carrying out a vaginal examination, or vulval inspection. A doctor might feel comfortable so long as a nurse is present through whom a patient of the opposite sex can be asked to undress: 'Sister, I would like to examine this lady/man', but would be rather less comfortable to have to say directly 'Please take off your shoes and pants for me to examine you.' A doctor's basic training might have made him comfortable with a patient of the opposite sex in the detached clinical atmosphere of a hospital, but he or she might feel less at ease in the patient's home, conducting an examination in the intimate aura of the patient's bedroom. Again, a doctor might feel reasonably comfortable carrying out physical examination on an ordinary patient, but be less at ease if the patient was also a social acquaintance or a colleague, because then it is more difficult to conduct the examination with the same impersonal clinical atmosphere.

If, in any of these circumstances, the doctor displays, either verbally or non-verbally, evidence of being even temporarily embarrassed, this feeling is likely to be conveyed to the patient and communication between them will inevitably be disrupted.

In other instances, the doctor's embarrassment may become apparent when the patient voices a sexual problem directly. If the doctor then attempts to evade the topic by responding negatively with something like 'You'll just have to learn to live with it' or 'Sex is not the most important thing in the world, especially at your time of life', or even to dismiss the matter brusquely with 'Well, you know what your husband is likely to do if you keep on refusing him', the patient will feel even more uncomfortable and unhappy, and will know better than to refer to the topic again.

Patients may also be discomforted if the doctor, in a misguided attempt to put them at ease, adopts a jocular familiarity. Some patients find this threatening, and it can inhibit communication, particularly on affective topics. But if the doctor maintains an unhesitating comfort—not distant and aloof, not familiar and threatening—this is communicated to the patient, making it much easier for him to talk about affective topics generally and certainly about sexual aspects of health.

THE PROBLEM OF THE DOCTOR'S ANXIETIES

Another group of factors that can inhibit communication on affective topics between patient and doctor are doctors' personal anxieties, arising in the context of their professional work. It is not very difficult for a student to recognize and understand how a *patient's* anxieties may influence the way he behaves. A similar mechanism can also affect doctors. Van Beukesom gave an excellent description of the influence of anxiety on doctor–patient communication [63]. Following his account, a doctor's anxieties are liable to extend into the three main areas detailed below.

Anxiety about inadequacy or failure

When embarking on the practice of medicine, young doctors naturally feel rather insecure, if only because of their lack of experience. Confidence in one's own professional skill and judgement grows gradually and at varying rates in different individuals, but some people compensate for the uncertainties of self-doubt and bolster a shaky confidence by adopting a rather pompous distant professional style. An authoritative, brusque manner can help to ensure that the doctor dominates the consultation, and makes it less likely that he is exposed to questioning that might reveal him not to be the clever, capable person he wishes to appear. As a consequence, he seems very unapproachable to the patient, and the aura of infallible competence that he carefully maintains makes it much more difficult for patients to expose *their* own emotional vulnerability to him.

It is easy for doctors to labour under the false belief that patients expect them *always* to have an answer to their problems and a cure for their ills. Of course, most doctors aspire to help their patients, and can therefore be reluctant to have to admit 'I don't know' or 'There is nothing more I can do' [64]. As Van Beukesom put it, doctors who adopt an aura of infallibility readily rationalize and justify their behaviour with assertions that 'The doctor must become the high-priest of modern times.' But doctors' professional wish not to fail their patients can unfortunately become a barrier to honesty, openness and, eventually, trust.

The student is wise to recognize that he will not, as a doctor, really be expected to be omnipotent and infallible. All the evidence shows that it is not on their omniscience that doctors' good reputation rests, or their protection from litigation lies. It is usually enough that they are seen to do their best, conscientiously and honestly. If, at times, this means that they must frankly admit the limitations of their medical prowess, at least they can do so in the knowledge that their reputation for approachability will be increased—a much more valuable asset in the long run.

Of course, it is easier for an *older* doctor to admit that he does not have an instant answer to every clinical problem. In an elderly doctor, this might be accounted evidence of his wisdom and maturity, whereas in a young doctor if could more readily be seen (and felt) as just a confession of inexperience or ignorance.

It is also not easy for a young doctor to reveal his vulnerability by admitting to the emotional stresses which his work involves. Medical training offers little guidance about how exposure to stress affects doctors and how to deal with its effects. As one student put it 'Doctors are not supposed to be vulnerable'.

Anxiety about patients' emotional reactions to sensitive topics. Breaking bad news

Doctors can feel seriously inhibited from mentioning topics that patients might be 'touchy' about, including such varied subjects as taking more responsibility for an ageing demented parent, previous termination of pregnancy, thoughts of suicide. Other questions that might need to be raised can be deeply resented and make the patient quite angry—matters such as infidelity, possible child abuse, homosexuality, the possibility that a skin rash might be factitious—to cite a few examples.

A student or less experienced doctor may not have learned the least upsetting ways of raising 'difficult' issues of this sort but, with or without this technical skill, may be desperately anxious not to provoke an angry scene. He may avoid this anxiety by never discussing 'personal', sensitive topics with patients.

Another emotional reaction from the patient that a doctor may fight shy of is the distress provoked by learning bad news. In an earlier section, we discussed how death and dying can be treated as topics too distressing to mention, though sometimes difficult to avoid. Doctors get considerable professional and personal satisfaction from being the bearers of good news (of cure, of recovery, of a problem resolved), but there are inevitably occasions when they must act as the bearers of bad news likely to cause emotional distress—tears, bewilderment, grief. They might have to tell someone that they are permanently and seriously disabled following injury; tell a couple that their infertility is absolute; tell a pregnant woman that her unborn infant has a major malformation. Because he is the bearer of the news, the doctor may, quite wrongly, feel blameworthy, and shrink from the task, or tackle it very awkwardly, feeling guilty about his impotence to help [65]. For some, the process of breaking bad news can feel like an unreal tragic play in which the doctor plays a part, assuming an empathic style while deep down feeling unmoved and aloof, though with an uneasy sense of emotional dishonesty. Such feelings of unreality may not be dissimilar to the patient's own feelings 'This cannot be true. It isn't really me they are talking about. Why don't I feel more upset by this terrible news?' For both doctor and patient, then, the reaction can be one of unreality, with suppressed emotion and avoidance of distress. If the doctor, unconsciously shielding himself from distress, becomes more than usually detached and formal, this aloofness is liable to appear to the patient as unsympathetic or even evasive. Many patients are themselves aware of the doctor's inner reluctance to break bad news, and sometimes may skate around direct questions which could require him to speak the truth. Equally, when bad news has been frankly conveyed, the patient often feels especially grateful, and develops much closer trust in the doctor. 'Thank you for being so frank with me. I'm sure it couldn't have been easy for you.'

Brewin [66] described three ways of giving bad news: the blunt, unfeeling way; the kind but sad and solemn way; and the (preferred) understanding, positive way. His paper is full of wise guidance, underlining the importance of observing and responding to the patient's reactions; of being truthful, but positive and hopeful; and of smiling to convey warmth and understanding.

It is helpful to keep in mind the following points. Vague or incomplete information with lack of detail increases uncertainty. As a result, anxiety grows and trust diminishes. Consider thoughtfully the information you need to give the patient. Reflect on what you might want to know if you were the patient, but keep in mind that we are all different. Do not attempt to rehearse the interview or stick to a line rigidly in the face of fresh cues from the patient as he or she takes in the news.

Many students and young doctors are fearful that they may face a torrent of questions and reactions for which they would be unprepared, and that they may then come out with inaccurate or inappropriate information. When reliable answers cannot be given, the doctor does best to acknowledge his uncertainty, and promise to raise the matter with the doctor in charge so that the patient can get an answer as soon as possible. When direct explicit questions are asked, only a truthful and forthright explanation of the facts is appropriate. Again, a subsequent interview with a more senior staff member can be offered, and patients encouraged to write down specific questions or concerns.

When breaking bad news, use simple lay terms, avoid jargon, and explain as precisely as possible the nature of the disease, the degree of seriousness, and the plan of management. Allow a liberal amount of silence between statements to provide an opportunity for questions and to encourage the expression of feelings. Offer to write down for the patient any necessary details if this seems appropriate, and be ready to go over the important facts more than once.

Avoid attempts to give a precise prognosis, since this is rarely accurate. By attempting not to raise false hopes, harm can result from undermining all hope. In the case of children and younger people, however, doctors are liable to be over-optimistic, and reluctant to divulge the seriousness of the situation.

The presence of a close relative or appropriate friend is desirable when serious news is to be conveyed. This helps to provide the patient with immediate support; it avoids the danger of a conspiracy of secrecy building up in the family; and it makes easier the recollection of what has been said. Useful feedback information can be obtained from relatives subsequently as to how much has been understood by the patient, and whether the interview achieved its objectives. If necessary, a second interview can then be helpful.

However bleak the prospects, the patient and family need to be reassured that, whatever complications arise, the medical and nursing teams will provide support throughout, and will do all in their power to minimize pain and distress. Some patients may be reluctant for the family to be told the seriousness of the situation. Explore why the patient does not wish to share this information, and indicate the problems likely to arise if the family are kept in the dark. Offer to be with the patient when the family are told, to help answer the questions that will inevitably ensue. The general practitioner is likely to be able to play a helpful part.

From the patient's point of view, the receipt of bad news is likely to come when they are at their most vulnerable. They are not just in need of reassurance, but utterly susceptible to any therapeutic suggestions from the doctor. Like a drowning man, they are ready to clutch at any straw. Obtaining consent to treatment at such a time requires additional care.

To improve the clarity of communication when breaking bad news to patients with cancer, Hogbin and Fallowfield [67] record each consultation on audiotape. They then give the cassette to the patient to take home, so that it is available for recap, and for other family members to hear.

A further kind of emotional 'scene' that a doctor may seek to avoid is any display of strife or discord, either involving himself or occurring between other people in his presence. His aversion to conflict and aggression may mean that he is unwilling to see together, let alone try to counsel, two people who are at odds with each other, such as an adolescent and a parent, a young woman and her mother-in-law, or a married couple whose relationship is under strain.

Anxiety relating to unresolved personal problems

An area of interpersonal conflict can create even more intense anxiety for a doctor if the difficulty in his patient's life mirrors some unresolved problem within his own personal and family life, some painful, distressing circumstance that he is trying to forget or keep out of his mind, or even to deny. There might, for example, be disharmony in his marriage; anxiety or conflict resulting from his adolescent children's experiments with sex, alcohol, or other drugs; guilt about an extramarital affair, or an abortion.

Because of deep sensitivity about such a topic, a doctor may bluntly brush off any discussion of a similar problem affecting one of his patients, or attempt to dismiss the whole matter with a joke:

'Look! I'm not a social worker. I'm a busy doctor.'

'I don't think I have time to go into that today.'

'Well. You've made your bed, you'll have to lie on it!'

We can therefore contrast the different influences a doctor's own experiences in life may have on his professional effectiveness. Sometimes the doctor's personal encounters with illness, disability, or emotional distress can provide him with great insight into patients' problems, and reinforce his ability to respond empathically to patients with similar misfortunes. If he gains the confidence to share his own experiences, this self-disclosure can promote strong mutual understanding (see p. 68). But if life has left him with tender emotional scars that have refused to heal, he may be professionally hamstrung when a patient presents with a comparable problem.

To summarize, the factors we have been discussing can and do have a big influence on doctors' professional manner. In different ways, they are liable to inhibit some doctors from involvement with affective aspects of ill health. Unless these inhibitions are understood, and neutralized through insight and professional skill, the doctor is likely to maintain a distance and a lack of warmth in his clinical work that he may not truly intend, but that constitute a barrier between himself and his patients through which he has no keys to pass.

No less unfortunately, these inhibitions are also liable to constrict the doctor's view of his patients. If the doctor is reluctant to talk about patients' close personal relationships, they are then likely to be perceived in isolation from the social context of their lives, and their illnesses.

This chapter has considered in some detail obstacles to communication which the doctor must learn to overcome. There are obstacles for the patient also. Timid patients will not reveal symptoms that they find embarrassing. Anxious patients may not disclose symptoms in case their worst fears might be realized. Unassuming patients will feel reluctant to mention complaints which they think would be dismissed as trivial, foolish, or inevitable—'only to be expected'. Elderly patients may be quite hesitant to complain of impairment of hearing, sight, urinary control, or memory.

Other aspects of doctor–patient communication

8

DECEPTIVE COMMUNICATION

Up to this point is has been tacitly assumed that communication between doctor and patient takes place 'on the level', that the exchanges are always characterized by honesty and openness. This is certainly not invariably the case, and sometimes lies or half-lies, deceptions, and denials are at the heart of the dialogue.

Deceit by the patient may take many forms, ranging from flagrant to subtle. Even the patient's initial complaints may be falsified. An unusual skin lesion (for example) may be factitious. Sometimes the motivation is obscure or psychopathic, as in Munchausen's syndrome (p. 8).

I recall an antenatal patient who remained in hospital for much of her pregnancy because of recurring episodes of bleeding. Whenever it was suggested that she might be discharged to her uncongenial home, she would retire (it came to light) to the toilet with her car keys and abrade her vaginal wall. Another patient, a nurse, was confined to bed with severe 'menorrhagia'. Because the flooding had evidently soaked through into her mattress, and because she evaded pelvic examination I suspected an incomplete abortion. In fact she had had a hysterectomy some years earlier, and the blood came from the pooled dregs of transfusion packs taken from the surgical ward where she worked!

An occasional patient may be malingering (oscillatory plumbism!) or seeking financial compensation for an alleged injury at work. Another may be concealing a secret about which he or she feels ashamed—drug misuse, child abuse, domestic violence, infidelity, or thoughts of suicide, for example. Sometimes the patient's motive may be to please, as much as to deceive the doctor. At post-operative follow-up, the insistent 'I'm feeling fine, doctor' may spring not from a sense of well-being, but from a desire not to disappoint the doctor (who has seemed to try so hard!) or just from dread that readmission to hospital or (worse) further surgery is a possibility. Lies about compliance in taking medication are common, and even written entries in (for example) diabetic diaries may be falsified. Patients with eating disorders (anorexia, bulimia,) are very likely to conceal their dietary compulsions.

While these are no more than a handful of examples of the ways in which the patient may set out to deceive the doctor, it is only fair to make clear that the doctor's professional command of the interview allows him to deceive the patient with much greater facility. A doctor's lapses into deceit could well involve information he presumes the patient may not wish to hear. He may feel that he is merely cloaking painful realities (in the case of a sinister diagnosis, for example) or diverting attention from the truth (when, say, the side-effects of treatment have become worse than the original complaint). The doctor's motive is often his aversion to uttering bad news. But half-truths and vagueness do not, in fact, always convince the patient, although the dust of pretence is likely to hang in the air and cloud the openness of the relationship.

COMMUNICATION WHEN THINGS GO WRONG

The circumstances described above are liable to occur in the course of everyday practice. But being less than honest has very different implications when things have gone wrong clinically. There might have been, for example, a toxic reaction to a drug, possibly following a prescribing error; an operative accident with visceral or vascular injury; a slipped ligature with a large haematoma. The patient and relatives, expecting an early recovery, are suddenly facing a relapse, or even the likelihood of death.

Unfortunately, the doctor's immediate reaction to the setback may to be clam up, or be evasive, perhaps distancing himself from the patient and relatives for a time and communicating only through intermediaries. Worst of all, he may try to lie his way out of trouble, or suggest that others are to blame. It is unwise to adopt a defensive posture, and to try to play down and dismiss patients' problems or criticisms. Be prepared, rather, to say 'Sorry', especially when the patient has sustained long-lasting or permanent harm.

As could be expected, the best prospect that the patient's confidence in the doctor will survive an upset of this sort is when good rapport has been maintained from the very first professional contact. Certainly, after a calamity or an error, openness is the wisest policy. The Medical Protection Society, in its annual report for 1990, gave the following guidance: 'The Society advocates a policy of full and proper communication with patients. In circumstances where complications or errors arise, it is proper that objective factual information, with appropriate clinical reassurance, is provided. Adequate explanation, ideally from the responsible consultant or principal, assists in reducing fear and uncertainty which may give rise to complaints and claims. The Society does not encourage members to withhold objective factual information.'

TALKING TO PEOPLE WITH A DISABILITY

Between those who regard themselves as 'normal' and those who are disabled, handicapped, or disfigured, there is undoubtedly an emotional divide, which can vitiate communication between 'them' and 'us'. Epilepsy, for example, has been described as 'a passport to prejudice—the only disorder where the patient is handicapped more by the attitude of society than by the disorder itself' [68].

Time of onset of disability

Some individuals are handicapped from birth. As in childhood they come to recognize their disabilities, they may feel isolated, marginalized, or belittled, and they often fear rejection because they are not perfect.

Others, previously able bodied, are overtaken at a later stage when in the full vigour of life by serious disability in various forms, such as spinal injury, multiple sclerosis, or renal failure. They mourn inwardly and bitterly that part of themselves that they have lost—the independence, sexual energy, or control of their lives. At the same time, they do not want to disappoint or appear unthankful to the doctors whose expertise has (perhaps) enabled them to survive, and who seem to *expect* them to be eternally grateful!

Others become disabled in their declining years, through stroke, hearing loss, Parkinson's disease, for example. They may feel they are becoming an undeserving burden on society, and so retain little sense of self-esteem or confidence in rehabilitation.

Disfigurement

A group of patients whose situation calls for the greatest sensitivity in communication are those disfigured by disease, accident, or the results of treatment. Even when the mutilation can be skilfully concealed (e.g. mastectomy, bowel stoma), its effect on the patient's sense of wholeness and sexual confidence may be devastating. Merely to ensure that the breast prosthesis or stoma bag is a perfect fit is not enough. The doctor needs to demonstrate the comfort (p.57) that will help the patient to express his or her painful feelings of loss of attractiveness with repelling barriers to intimacy.

Other disfigurements, such as generalized skin disease (eczema, psoriasis, vitiligo in those with dark skins), cannot be concealed. Those which affect the facial appearance are likely to cause the most distress, whether they result from birth defects, scars, acne, or other conditions. Such patients are liable to become socially withdrawn, and may shrink into reclusive isolation. Although sometimes a doctor may feel that a particular patient is over-reacting to a comparatively minor problem, he should avoid any attempt to trivialize the patient's concern. Dismissive remarks such as 'I've seen many cases much worse than this' or 'It's the sort of scarring that will gradually fade with time'. are likely to alienate rather than reassure the patient. In the final analysis, only the individual affected can appraise the significance of a perceived disfigurement. Whatever causes distress cannot be disregarded as trifling. This applies to problems in adolescents such as facial acne or hypertrophic pendulous breasts, and to alopecia or excessive facial hair in women.

Patients with transplants

These patients can have difficulty in communicating their concerns to their doctors. They are liable to side-effects from immunosuppressive drugs, such as weight gain, pallid loose skin ('You look awful!'), aching bones, debilitating lethargy, periods of insomnia, loss of sex drive. But the patients do not want to let down those whose skills have enabled them to survive, so they hesitate to voice their negative feelings and unpleasant complaints to the staff. The doctors equally tend to act as if the patients ought to be eternally grateful for their technical brilliance, and may be inclined to respond grudgingly to patients' complaints and queries, and sense of loss—'Somehow, I'm not whole any more. I just feel powerless'.

The feelings which can be evoked by those who are regarded as other-than-normal may fluctuate between embarrassment, aversion, pity, and dread. At the same time their recurrent frustration because of their disabilities, and irritation because of others' attitudes towards them, can at times find expression in aggressive and angry behaviour, with stubborn unco-operative reactions. They may resent the use of terms such as handicapped, affliction, or victim. Therefore, it is perhaps not surprising that normal dialogue is liable to be distorted in a variety of ways. Some of the potential sources of misunderstanding or antagonism are discussed below.

Patronizing

The disabled person is at risk of being talked down to, or patronized in other ways. He may be addressed with slow speech in a rather loud voice, as though, like a child, he couldn't easily grasp what is said. He may be offered extravagant praise: 'It's wonderful that he manages to do so much! These people are marvels—a lesson to us all!'

Although disability and dependence may tend to bring out the worst aspects of the doctor's paternalism ('Doctor knows best!'), in fact many people with a disability are driven to acquire an enhanced degree of self-reliance and expertise in coping with their problem. They are therefore likely to be suspicious or hypercritical towards strange or inexperienced health workers, preferring to place their confidence in only one or two trusted attendants. To quote Hughes [69]: 'If we could learn the secret of coping with illhealth which some of our patients possess, but which to others proves so elusive, the discovery would be infinitely more worthwhile than the most specific monoclonal antibody.'

As a first step towards better rapport with those people who have disabilities, the learner can generate more confidence by acknowledging his own need to learn rather than by proffering solutions—'Look, I'll have to learn from you how this condition affects your life. Can you tell me how you tackle the problems your disability causes?'

Ignoring

At worst, the patient with a disability may not be just talked down to, but talked over. Enquiries and remarks are addressed to a third party, an attendant or relative, and the patient is ignored. There is no direct vocal or eye contact. This disastrous scenario is epitomized in the enquiry 'Does he take sugar?'

Jocularity

It is common for people generally, and doctors no less, to attempt to mask feelings of awkwardness by recourse to jocularity. 'You'll have to fit either a horn or a tachograph on that wheelchair!' This sort of jocular approach is likely to be perceived as insensitive or even offensive.

Demeaning

Despite their wish to be treated like anyone else, and their (usual) preference for the company of non-disabled people, the disabled tend to become isolated during everyday social discourse, or even segregated in certain settings. Because their circle of friends is constricted and their confidants few, they are inclined to feel shy and awkward in company.

As an unfortunate extension of this apartness, and because they are other than normal in various respects (behaviour, appearance, etc.) disabled people may be treated in subtle ways as somehow less than human, in terms of their personal dignity, and the respect and independence they are afforded. Even the way of thinking about, and lumping together 'the disabled' or 'the handicapped' as a group sets them apart from us, who think of ourselves as 'normal' human beings. We can help to restore the sense of individuality and dignity by not only treating each patient as a person, but also by recognizing his or her disabilities as individual—as particular to one person.

Every effort therefore needs to be made to try to ensure that the disabled can take as much independent control of their lives as possible, particularly in hospitals or other institutions. When they are offered assistance, either physical or otherwise, it should be done with tact, avoiding the presumption that they are helpless or inept. During undressing and dressing (perhaps awkwardly) their privacy needs to be carefully protected. Again, if they need help, it should be offered without loss of dignity. Their sexual feelings, which tend to be ignored, need to be acknowledged, and their expression regarded as natural and, where necessary, facilitated.

TALKING ABOUT PAIN

Acute pain is a common symptom of the onset of illness. If the doctor listens carefully, the patient's description of the nature of the pain will often help to reveal the diagnosis. The time of onset, the site (and possible shifting) of the pain, the verbal description—stabbing, crushing, nagging, agonizing, niggling, colicky, tearing, steady, unremitting—all convey important information. This is in large measure because acute pain is usually nociceptive in type, and noxious stimuli can be closely correlated with the disease process or injury that has activated them.

However, the pathophysiology of much chronic pain is uncertain. It may be nociceptive in type; or neuropathic; or psychogenic; or any combination of these. To complicate matters further, there is often a circular interaction involving chronic pain, via disability, inactivity, distress, fear, and despair. These factors can exacerbate the patient's perception of the pain, leading to depression (see also p.101). Chronic pain in some locations—facial pain, lower abdominal pain in women, ill-localized backache—is notoriously difficult to characterize.

When there is an apparent disparity between the objective clinical findings and the patient's declared disability, the possibility of malingering or compensation-seeking has to be considered. Sometimes the complaint of pain is perpetuated because the patient has become dependent on analgesic drugs.

PALLIATIVE CARE

The recent recognition accorded to the new specialty of palliative care is an indication that particular skills are required in this area of practice. The doctors and other professionals concerned have discarded the claim to control the course of disease. Their relationship with patients is based not on the authority to heal and restore, but on openness and honesty, which can be no less potent in generating trust. At the same time, they are using their skills to sustain the quality of life for the patient to the end of the road. These attitudes can be contrasted with what Weatherall [70] has called 'modern high-technology patch-up practice' where 'patients are liable to be pushed to the extremes of their endurance by the most intensive protocols of chemotherapy, some of which require them to be taken to Death's door in an attempt to eradicate their tumours.'

In the task of caring rather than attempting to cure, a team of professionals is involved. The doctor therefore does not hold centre stage, but other carers, such as MacMillan nurses, contribute vital skills. Importantly, the members of the team provide one another with professional support, and so reduce the stresses of their task. Communication skills are central in work of this sort, which is dealt with in more detail in Chapter 12.

Testing topics

M.J. FORD

TALKING ABOUT PSYCHOSOMATIC ILLNESS

At least one-third of all patients referring themselves to a general practitioner or presenting to a general medical clinic have no evidence of underlying organic disease to account for their symptoms. They do not have frank psychiatric illness, and are conventionally considered to have functional disorders. The term 'functional disorder' is, unfortunately, sometimes used in a pejorative or dismissive manner, as biomedical science has become the focus of medical attention.

Altered emotional states are commonly associated with physical symptoms, and most people will have experienced (say) urinary frequency before an interview or an examination. Some individuals do not find it easy to admit to, much less to express, the emotions which are disturbing them; others lack the insight and emotional vocabulary which would help them to associate their physical symptoms with an emotional problem. As Balint [124] has said, some illnesses allow patients to complain of a problem.

A few doctors see their role within the restricted focus of the biomedical realm, and consider that the exclusion of underlying organic disease is all that is required of them. Identification of relevant psycho-social influences is considered by them to be the responsibility of other 'better-trained' doctors such as general practitioners or psychiatrists. Those doctors who feel ill at ease dealing with patients who have no physical stigmata of disease cope with this situation better if they can be dismissed as either psychiatrically ill or malingering.

At the same time, inexperienced young clinicians can feel considerable anxiety when dealing with patients whose symptoms they are unable to explain. If this anxiety is transmitted back to the patient, the end result may be to stimulate continuing fruitless investigations, aimed to exclude increasingly remote and unlikely diagnoses. It is regrettable that some physicians feel more concern that they might overlook organic disease than that they fail to identify significant psychosocial stress or emotional morbidity.

If the physician is conditioned to assume that every bona fide patient must have an organic disease, and if none is discovered, the doctor may oscillate uneasily between two alternatives: either organic disease has been missed, or the patient needs psychiatric referral. If then the pathway of over-zealous investigation is followed, this can powerfully reinforce the patient's anxieties, and perpetuate or localize previously vague and transient symptoms.

It is therefore wise to review the patient with persistent symptoms but negative findings before embarking on anxiety-provoking and potentially hazardous further investigations. The presence or absence of changes in symptoms and signs can be a helpful diagnostic pointer. The review needs to encompass all aspects of the patient's personal situation, and any current or past sources of emotional stress.

Every effort should be made to establish the diagnosis of a functional disorder in a positive way, rather than merely by a process of exclusion. Some patients have personality traits in which the amplification of physical symptoms is a repeated characteristic; some may be responding to life events or difficult relationships; others may have no evident immediate explanation for their symptoms.

Pain is a common presenting symptom of psychosomatic illness and, as a subjective experience, it may be difficult to evaluate. Attempts to distinguish between real and imaginary pain are unhelpful, and made more difficult by virtue of the influence of personality and mood on the perception of pain. Pain may dominate the clinical picture so completely that the emotional state becomes difficult to assess, and the patient is unable to recognize feelings of anxiety or depression.

Some somatic complaints are amplifications of normal physiological sensations. If a patient complains of symptoms which are widely prevalent normally, and which do not usually precipitate requests for consultation, the implication is that there are factors rendering the patient less able to tolerate such sensations. It can be more relevant to ask why people behave in this way than to ask what is wrong with them.

The 'sick role'

A better understanding of some functional conditions can be reached using the concepts of the 'sick role' and illness behaviour. Being regarded as sick carries with it certain privileges. In addition to the exemption from everyday responsibilities, there is an implicit obligation on others to be kind and sympathetic to the sick, as well as to relieve them of their normal duties. The only obligation of being a patient is to seek and accept treatment, so that the privileges of the sick role are claimed for as short a time as possible. Individuals who behave as if they were ill when the demands of everyday life become excessive may do so because they have experienced gain from this behaviour in the past.

There is considerable overlapping between organic illness, illness engendered by fear of ill health, and illness induced by the rewards of the sick role. The philosophical dualism of Cartesian metaphysics—the neat separation of mind and body—has little relevance in the practice of medicine, where the two are firmly integrated, and where boundaries therefore overlap.

There are wider dimensions to every illness experience, which determine how patients perceive, interpret, and react to bodily changes. Personal psycho-social factors may, at one extreme, account for the denial of illness, and at the other for requests for consultation disproportionate to the severity of the illness. A small minority of patients may adopt the sick role semi-permanently if they experience the normal demands of life as excessive, either because they lack the resolve to cope, or because only when ill do they receive sufficient sympathy and attention. In the majority, however, the sick role only becomes attractive when adversity is abnormally great, perhaps at a time of severe stress with exacerbation of chronic anxiety. Since it is usually difficult or impossible to separate conscious from unconscious motivation, it is counter-productive to insinuate that symptoms are not totally genuine, particularly as the patients concerned may themselves have doubts about this. The wiser approach is to emphasize that the symptoms are very familiar, that serious illness has been safely excluded, and that significant improvement can be expected.

Varieties of psychosomatic disorder

Psychosomatic disorders are, by their very nature, protean in their expression. They vary also from one culture to another. But they cannot escape from being labelled and categorized. The medical axiom that diagnosis must precede treatment is deeply rooted in medical thinking. It is a commendable principle, even though it can lure doctors into unreasonable investigations in the search for diagnostic certainty, or into earnest but esoteric debate about taxonomic niceties. A diagnostic label not only provides the doctor with a convenient handle, but also conveys assurance that a diagnosis has been achieved. Patients too are often relieved to learn that their illness has a name, with the assumption that the doctor now knows what is wrong!

Diagnostic labels come and go as fashions change. Shell-shock, effort syndrome, and neurasthenia are now historical; irritable bowel syndrome, chronic fatigue syndrome, and post-traumatic stress disorder are examples of current labelling.

While accepting the overlapping of boundaries already referred to, broad but recognizable categories of psychosomatic disorders are encountered.

Pathophysiological reactions

Emotional distress produces characteristic physical symptoms, including lack of energy, headaches, sleep disturbance, altered sexual function, anorexia, constipation, diarrhoea, and altered bladder function. Most individuals are familiar with a tension headache. Disorders associated with exaggerated reactions to stress include the irritable bowel syndrome, asthma, hypertension, and many others. Anxiety states and panic disorders commonly provoke hyperventilation, with symptoms attributable to the over-breathing.

Amplification of normal body sensations

Stress can enhance the perception of physiological phenomena. For example, palpitation may be experienced during periods of anxiety without any change in heart rhythm.

Hypochondriasis

A recurrent and firmly held conviction of having, or a fear of having serious illness is an essential hallmark of hypochondriacal disorders. When the condition comes on for the first time in later life, however, depressive illness should be suspected.

Conversion disorder

Abrupt alteration or loss of bodily function in response to acute psychological stress in the absence of organic disease is the typical feature. Previously known as hysteria, the condition usually arises in young adults.

Somatoform pain disorder

The condition is characterized by preoccupation with persistent pain which is disproportionate to or unaccompanied by underlying organic disease.

Somatization disorders

These are characterized by multiple physical complaints, which cannot be explained on the basis of organic disease. The history often originates in childhood or young adulthood.

Patients with somatization disorders are less likely than others to recognize or even accept the possibility that physical symptoms may be related to emotional problems. Indeed, such patients may interrupt the doctor's attempt at an exposition of the problem with an interjection such as 'I suppose you think it's all in my mind?' Such a response may be conveying a number of messages, of the patient's own anxiety about whether or not the symptoms are real; about whether or not the physician believes the account of the illness; and about concern that any admission of emotional distress would in some way undermine the validity of the symptoms to such an extent that the physician would not investigate further.

What to tell the patient

The care of patients with psychosomatic disorders needs to include continuing reassurance that, even if a diagnosis cannot be made with absolute certainty, serious disease can be safely excluded on clinical grounds. This reassurance is more likely to be effective if it follows a careful review of symptoms both physical and emotional, and a thorough physical examination. When symptoms cannot be readily explained after organic disease has been excluded, it is often wiser to admit this defeat than to invent implausible explanations which fail to satisfy the patient. It can be particularly helpful to elicit and discuss patients' own concept of their illness, and to what they attribute their symptoms. Empathy is important in management, helping to assure the patient that the symptoms are regarded as real, though enigmatic.

Even though some patients will not accept a psychological explanation for their symptoms, a consistent supportive approach, with the offer of further appointments, is important. A long-term relationship with a single clinician (ideally the general practitioner) should help to discourage 'doctor shopping' and the inappropriate involvement of multiple specialists.

THE DIFFICULT DOCTOR–PATIENT RELATIONSHIP

Notions of the 'good doctor' and the 'good patient' are firmly entrenched and difficult to brush aside. The idealized good doctor is omniscient and all-powerful; always pleasant, always present, attentive, perceptive, and empathic. He avoids confrontation and skilfully empowers patients, allowing them to make their own decisions and take responsibility over their own health This ideal doctor is quick to listen and slow to judge. Intimate and paternalistic when the need arises, he nevertheless encourages patients to maintain autonomy and individualism. Deeply self-aware, such a doctor is able to tune into an infinite range of patients, their personalities, and their family members.

Stereotypical good patients are articulate, but brief and precise. They always arrive five minutes before any appointment, and dress in such a way as to facilitate speedy examination. They are always scrupulously clean and smell sweetly. Such patients are keen to hand over responsibility for the interview, their illnesses, and their lives to the doctor. They always accept advice and never give it. They follow all instructions to the letter, and quickly change those habits which have led to ill health or which exacerbate symptoms.

Clearly, these stereotypes are unreal, and rarely encountered in the flesh. Some of these idealized attributes are mutually exclusive. For instance, the doctor must be able to confront key issues with the patient as much as the patient must be able to express their true feelings if they are to participate actively in difficult medical decisions. Doctors cannot be loved and respected by all of their patients all of the time, nor can they expect of themselves an ability to warm towards all of their patients. When problems arise, therefore, it is important to consider: Whose problem is it, the patient's or the doctor's? Why are both doctor and patient behaving as they do? What has gone wrong between them, and how best can the doctor establish or restore a better relationship?' If, in the jargon of commerce, the customer is always right, it may be wiser to start from the assumption that the patient is right. In many instances the irritating patient can equally be seen as a reflection of an irritable doctor, and so the key to a better understanding of such patients is a better understanding of ourselves.

Difficult doctor–patient relationships can arise in a number of scenarios:

Patient factors
- Dirty, unkempt, or smelly patients
- Deceiptful or evasive patients
- Patients who abuse alcohol or other drugs.
- Patients who formally complain about their treatment,
- Hostile and/or litigious patients.
- Manipulative or sexually provocative patients.
- 'Ungrateful' patients who never admit to feeling better.
- Obsessive patients preoccupied with minutiae of their illness.

Doctor factors
- Rude, overbearing, and inconsiderate doctors.
- Doctors experiencing emotional distress or physical exhaustion through lack of sleep, overwork, etc.
- Doctors with difficulties in their personal lives—relationships, alcohol, etc.

- Doctors developing mental illness.

- Doctors over extended professionally, beyond their training and capabilities.

- Doctors lacking a confidant or other professional support.

- Doctors with conflicting interests—ethical, managerial, commercial.

When the expectations of the patient and the doctor are at variance, conflict is liable to arise. Such a clash of expectations, often implicit but unstated, commonly relates either to problems of sharing power within the interplay of the relationship, or to behavioural divergencies between the doctor and patient.

A relationship is particularly likely to be difficult when the doctor is assuming conflicting roles. This could arise when looking after close friends or relatives, a fellow physician, or when either doctor or patient is aware of sexual attraction between them. Similarly, difficulty can arise when there is a potential ethical conflict, as when doctors undertake insurance medical examinations acting on behalf of a company rather than the patient. The interests of the two parties are often diametrically opposed. Many doctors are now increasingly responsible for resource management and its optimal utilization. Thus, they may be drawn into the role of gatekeeper, barring access to to more expensive investigations or treatments. When wearing such a hat in addition to a clinical hat, conflicts of interest are very likely to occur.

Other examples of ethical difficulty include the prescription of addictive drugs to patients thought to be habituated; prescribing contraceptives to underage teenagers; and the issues surrounding abortion. Further examples are the treatment of individuals whose health is impaired by the abuse of tobacco, alcohol, or other drugs.

Conflicts of interest can also occur when, during clinical care, the doctor would like to recruit the patient into a research project, the purpose of which will have little or no direct benefit for the individual concerned, and may expose him to significant hazard. Finally, another common area of conflict arises when patients request certification for days off work, or for compensation claims for illnesses which the doctor adjudges are either trivial or factitious.

Strategies for coping

Although individual doctors and patients are all different, some general strategies are useful when faced with a difficult doctor–patient relationship. First, look within youself and ask 'What is it about me that finds this situation/patient so irritating? Do the patient and I share similar sensitivities and frailties?' Seeing our own flaws in others can arouse intolerance. Understanding why one is so 'allergic' to a certain patient's behaviour may help not only at the time, but also in avoiding similar difficult relationships in the future.

Only after this introspective exercise should one move on to consider 'What is it about this patient that irritates me?' While observing the bounds of confidentiality, share your feelings with a professional colleague or close confidant. Remember that when a consultation goes badly in a busy clinic, it can have a knock-on effect during subsequent consultations. This makes it particularly helpful to ventilate one's feelings after the patient has left the consulting room.

When genuine conflict is arising, make an effort to re-establish more effective rapport with the patient. Try to clearly identify and acknowledge the nature of the conflict as explicitly as possible with the patient: 'Look, we seem to be in danger of falling out over this question of . . .'

If there is an issue about the assumption of responsibilities, it may help to negotiate explicit responsibilities for both patient and doctor, keeping the patient's concerns in mind, and occasionally even drawing up a written mutually agreed contract, defining what responsibilities each will carry. Review the agreed plan of management regularly with the patient, to ensure that both parties are fulfilling their commitments.

For example, many doctors find communication with young people addicted to drugs very difficult, and may respond by avoiding all such contacts, and declining to be involved in their care. These patients are then shuffled around from practitioner to practitioner, a movement often accelerated by frequent conflicts. In such a situation, it is better to explain to the patient the difficulties you find in sharing responsibility for the care of an addict. After agreeing a firm contract of responsibilities and duties, as discussed, make explicit your expectations of the patient's behaviour, i.e. in the waiting room they must not be abusive or physically thretening to fellow patients or staff; they must not make out of hours calls for the supply of drugs; they must not distribute to their friends any drugs supplied to them. In return, the doctor will prescribe a specific quantity of drugs each week, with no replacement of 'lost' prescriptions. Breaking the agreement will result in the patient being asked to seek another practitioner. This sort of contract can help to avoid the anger generated by an adversarial approach.

DEALING WITH ANGRY PATIENTS AND RELATIVES

Anger arises in many instances as a response to loss or the threat of loss. The loss may be real, for instance the death of a loved one, or may be perceived, i.e. the threat of loss of dignity or self-esteem. To take a common example, patients can become intensely irritated if their appointment with the doctor is delayed, and they have to wait unexpectedly. Some may feel impelled to complain angrily on behalf of a less articulate patient, such as a child or elderly relative. Often, the trigger to anger is disproportionately small compared to the response evoked, and there may be little clear relationship between the triggering event and the emotive response. It is important, therefore, always to consider the possibility of a hidden cause, i.e. a simmering emotion which is finding an outlet as anger about being kept waiting. The patient may feel that not to complain would indicate a weakness of character. For some, the act of complaining is so stressful that it cannot be tackled without building up a pressure head of anger.

A golden rule when dealing with anger or angry complaints is to be quick to listen and slow to judge. Try to acknowledge that the patient's feelings of anger are understandable. 'I can see that you feel very angry. If you have been waiting so long, you have every right to feel like that. I am very sorry that you have been kept waiting. I shall try to do everything in my power to minimize any further delay.'

When you sense that the patient is angry but not overtly so, try to elicit and identify the feeling. 'You look upset. What has happened to upset you? Are you feeling angry?' Then pause in silence. This will allow the patient to either admit or deny the anger, and to give voice to their feelings. Be slow to judge, and try to understand how the patient is feeling, why they feel angry, where they think the blame lies, and how they feel the matter should be handled. Above all, help them to take control of the situation while showing acceptance, empathy, and support. If the patient cannot propose a solution to the problem, suggest the options open to them. Resist the temptation to suppress the emotion, or to divert it, unless the intensity of the anger or the patient's personality suggests that violence is likely to be imminent. In such an event, placate the individual and unobtrusively call for help.

TALKING WITH RELATIVES

The consent of the patient is necessary before disclosing any medical information to a relative. This important consideration can easily be overlooked when a relative happens to come across the doctor unexpectedly, perhaps in the course of attending another clinic or ward. It is therefore helpful when talking with patients to remember to seek their views as to how much information should be made available to family members. If this is done routinely, the possibility of a breach of confidentiality is minimized.

In prearranged interviews with family members, it is very useful to ensure, if possible, that the patient is present throughout the interview, and is kept in the forefront of the ensuing discussion. The tendency to overlook the patient when discussing matters raised by the family members—the 'Does he take sugar?' syndrome—must be avoided. Patients with communication difficulties, particularly the elderly with deafness or dementia, or patients with language difficulty necessitating the use of an older child as interpreter, produce situations which require handling with special tact and sensitivity.

If the patient can be encouraged to control the interview and to be the intermediary through whom questions are asked and to whom answers are addressed, the patient is unlikely to be sidelined. A number of common scenarios illustrate various issues:

'I hope you don't mind me speaking to you, doctor, but dad and I are very close. If there is something serious wrong with him, it is very important that he never finds out the truth. Otherwise he just couldn't cope.' Faced with this invitation to participate in a collusion of deceipt, it can be helpful to put to the family members how they might feel in their dad's shoes, if the rest of the family were trying to keep a painful truth from them. In this sort of situation, no rigid policy is likely to be universally helpful. An approach tailored to the needs of each patient and family should be the aim, with the patient's 'right to know' always given due weight.

The care of an elderly relative may precipitate another type of problem interview. All too often, the burden of care and responsibility has fallen upon one particular member of the family, who feels increasingly oppressed by the situation and unable to cope much longer.

'Doctor, I wonder if I could have a word with you about my mother? Over the last year things have been getting more and more difficult, as I have not been keeping well myself. *Something must be done about mum!*'

If the patient cannot return home in the absence of the daughter's support, and will continue to occupy a hospital bed, the doctor is liable to react judgementally to these remarks. This in turn may make the daughter feel even more put on. Suggest to the daughter that the conversation could be even more useful with mother present. Try to appreciate the daughter's perspective and encourage the patient, as appropriate, to take control and express her feelings and preferred solutions. In many instances, elderly patients much prefer to take their chance living in a precarious situation at home, rather than abandoning their autonomy and submitting themselves to nursing home care. If it is impractical for the patient either to live at home or to be looked after by a family member, a sensitive but realistic exposition of the options available to the patient and her family is necessary. Encourage the patient to negotiate a solution which, if not shared by all, can be understood and accepted by all.

DEALING WITH COMPLAINTS

When complaints arise, it is wise to assume, whatever the circumstances, that a failure in communication may well have contributed to the problem. Doctors and nurses are not infallible, and it is inevitable that mistakes, usually but not always minor, will occur from time to time. Fear of the consequences if and when the full facts emerge tends to provoke denial, and delay in responding to the complaint. In addition, the loss of self-esteem and the self-doubt which is liable to arise following a mistake can influence the way the complaint is handled. (See also p. 90).

There is no medico-legal reason why a doctor should not apologize promptly and unreservedly when a justifiable complaint is received, and try to explain the details and circumstances surrounding the incident to the patient and family. In many instances this prompt response may avert legal involvement.

When a patient or relatives complain, it is first necessary to establish from all those involved the facts of the matter. This allows the patient and family to be given a timely explanation of what happened and why, together with an apology as appropriate. It is vital to listen carefully to the complaint, and so try to appreciate the patient's feelings and perspective about what has gone wrong. After a mistake, the patient is liable to feel a powerless victim. Try to restore the patient's sense of control by giving over the lead and seeking their views on how best the matter can be resolved. Even when the problem has arisen from a fault of the system rather than of any single individual, a sincere apology is still fitting, together with an expression of intent to avoid similar occurrences in the future.

Again, the temptation to stifle or deflect any emotional responses during the interview must be resisted, and the patient and family given the opportunity to ventilate their feelings. If possible, try to negotiate a solution which both parties find acceptable. If the matter remains unresolved, discuss it without delay with a senior colleague. This should help to lessen your own anxiety, and may point towards an appropriate solution. If legal involvement appears likely or inevitable, make sure there is a clear detailed record of the events and difficulties surrounding the matters at issue, together with notes of any interviews.

PATIENT EDUCATION

Before a consultation concludes, a clear explanation of the problem, differential diagnosis (if any), and proposed treatment options should be made so that the patient fully understands the position. This so-called 'exposition' requires due consideration and adequate time within the framework of the clinical interview. Focus on the essential points, and emphasize these by repetition, avoiding the use of medical jargon. To check that the patient has grasped the information correctly, it is useful to ask the patient how they would explain their problem to another member of the family.

In this context it can be helpful to provide written instructions and relevant pamphlets covering the patient's disorder and its management in order to reiterate the information. The ideal practice is to arrange that a copy of the post-consultation letter to the general practitioner is also sent to the patient at home, so that both have received the same information. Make sure also that there is an agreed follow-up plan, and enquire whether the patient foresees any difficulty in complying with therapy, and how the doctor might best help the patient's efforts.

Two key questions are: 'What does the patient want to know?' and 'What does the patient need to know?' Ask the patient what further information they would like, and what questions for them or their family remain unanswered. Take time to explain the significance of symptoms and signs, and the results of investigations. Invite the patient to take responsibility for the necessary changes in lifestyle to prevent progression or recurrence of illness, and encourage the patient in this effort. Make sure also that the patient understands the nature and possible side-effects of any drug therapy, what to look for and how to respond in the event of an adverse reaction. Enquire if the patient is anxious at the prospect of taking a drug; explore any other potential problems of drug compliance for any other reason.

For many patients, ill health is made significantly worse by problems arising from lifestyle, difficult interpersonal relationships, and the abuse of alcohol, tobacco, and other drugs. Although a few may stop smoking in response to brief advice or a physician's lecture on the habit, most will not. When behavioural changes are desirable, try to help the individual patient to identify which behavioural change is most likely to result in better health, and which they feel most motivated to tackle. For instance, an obese patient with a major alcohol problem who is also a heavy smoker, presenting with recurrent pancreatitis, would be best advised to address the alcohol problem before considering trying to stop smoking, and a significant reduction in alcohol intake would also result in a fall in weight. Be realistic. Elderly patients who are lifelong smokers may have little to gain from stopping smoking, especially if they are asymptomatic.

If the doctor is to be helpful in effecting or at least catalysing behavioural change, such as stopping smoking, a good rapport and alliance with the patient is essential. Identify the factors which have induced the patient to continue the health-threatening behaviour, and stress the positive benefits to be gained by stopping. Help the patient to recognize the opportunity to quit and to seize the moment, even if there have been previous unsuccessful attempts. Secure as much support for the patient as possible, to reinforce their efforts. This may mean enlisting the support of a partner, or of a self-help group. Help the patient develop a plan and time-scale for change, and explore with them how to cope with initial lack of success. Be encouraging and reassuring. Commit yourself to an explicit plan for follow-up to reaffirm your interest in helping the patient towards a goal.

10 Talking about choices and making decisions

We now turn to the latter part of a medical interview, during which the doctor usually needs to outline the options open to the patient, and steer the dialogue towards decision-making. Often therefore this is the crux of the whole interview and sometimes it provides the greatest test of the doctor's skill as a communicator.

This part of the interview has been called 'the exposition', because traditionally the doctor was expected to pronounce, with all his professional authority, his views and conclusions about the diagnosis and to spell out what should be done. The phrase 'doctor's orders' (implying in general usage unquestioned authority) reflects the passive acceptance which was expected from patients. Similarly, the terms 'prescription' and 'compliance' carry the same authoritarian overtones.

But before framing, let alone voicing, his own conclusions, the doctor should always keep in mind the following two central questions:

Why has the patient come?

In some consultations certain patients will indeed expect from the doctor nothing more than the briefest of expositions—a diagnosis (possibly); a prescription and brief instructions; a reassuring phrase of dismissal, such as 'You'll soon be well again!'

But other patients have quite different expectations from the consultation. Some of them may have little interest in receiving a diagnostic label or even treatment, but only want some particular reassurance, for example:

- that they have not got cancer (or some other feared disease);

- that they do not need an operation or admission to hospital, and can continue the normal pattern of their life;

- that they *do* have a physical disorder and that their symptoms are not all imagined ('I was beginning to think it was all in my mind, doctor. I am so relieved!');

- that what is happening to them is to be expected in (for example) old age or pregnancy or the menopause or during fatigue or temporary stress—it is 'normal';

- that their symptoms are not going to get worse and become disabling.

Some patients, in contrast, are insistent above all that the consultation should provide them with a diagnostic label, to justify their continuing in a protected or dependent sick role, with avoidance of work or other obligations. They are therefore also likely to be averse to any therapeutic suggestions. Others wear their diagnosis as some sort of proud badge—'The professor said mine was the biggest ulcer/worst case he'd ever seen!'

Others again may be indifferent about either diagnosis or therapy, but only want from the consultation a sympathetic listening ear and a little encouragement. In return for saying almost nothing, doing nothing but listening attentively, the doctor will be thanked for 'being so helpful'.

What does the patient want?

The second and all important question concerns the patient's wishes. Making choices and decisions can at times require sensitive counterbalancing of relative advantages and disadvantages, of possible risks and benefits, of potential gains and losses. Sometimes ethical attitudes and philosophical values are also involved in the assessment of options (see below). In this complex process it is the *patient*'s views that are all important, if not paramount. However clear-cut the doctor's judgement about the action that needs to be taken, it is the patient who really must decide. Without his active consent and co-operation, confidence and compliance are unlikely to be forthcoming.

There are, however, limits to the patient's autonomy. (See also p. 129). It does not include the right to choose to die, nor the right to decide independently when resuscitation or life support for a close relative should be abandoned. The High Court ruled in 1992 that an anorexic teenager whose life was thought to be in danger did not have the right to refuse treatment. Similarly, parents do not (always) have autonomous choice in decisions about their own children, even when strongly held religious convictions are involved, for example in the case of Jehovah's Witnesses and Christian Scientists.

UNDERSTANDING CHOICES AND DECISIONS

Just as the initial part of the interview is more effectively handled with a grasp of the underlying diagnostic reasoning (p. 26), so the latter part of the consultation needs to be conducted with an understanding of the issues involved in medical decision-making. What is implied by informed consent, and to what extent is it an attainable goal? What are the proper limits of the doctor's 'authority' and the patient's 'autonomy'? If the doctor's and the patient's scale of values are not the same, how are they likely to differ, and how can they best be reconciled?

Informed consent

However acquiescent patients may have been expected to be in the past, in contemporary practice many patients expect to be given a full account of their condition and to be asked for their consent in all decisions relating to their health. This is a natural consequence of better public education about health, and of prevailing social attitudes about the autonomy of the individual.

These changes in public expectations are reflected in the Guidance on Patient Consent issued by the Department of Health in 1990 [71], and the Patients Charter 1991 [72]. The guidance notes set out clearly that the patient has a fundamental right to grant or withhold consent prior to examination or treatment; that the patient has a right to an explanation of investigation, treatment or operation, in terms suited to the understanding of the patient (parent or guardian); that the consent of the child *and* the parent or guardian should be obtained to treat children under the age of 16, except in an emergency. The doctor has to assess whether the child is competent to give informed consent. Children are entitled to refuse if they have sufficient understanding to make informed decisions. Competence to make an informed decision is generally a relevant issue in the case of children, the very elderly, the mentally ill, those with learning disabilities, those extremely anxious or shocked, and those speaking through an interpreter. There are, of course, important medico-legal reasons why doctors always need to secure written evidence of informed consent for operative procedures. Informed consent and the patient's 'right to know' are not, however, basic doctrines of British law. The legal standard of adequacy of the information given to patients in Britain is that of 'generally approved medical practice', i.e. what a 'responsible body of medical opinion' would regard as acceptable practice. As Law Lord Scarman has commented, it leaves unaddressed the question of what an average patient would wish to know. It is generally considered that patients should be made aware of substantial or special risks when treatments are offered. As an ideal or goal, informed consent is an admirable principle. But it is prudent to consider what are its limitations in practical terms, given that it is the doctor, during the exposition, who is the main source of the information on which the patient's choices rely.

Some limitations of informed consent

Patient's decisions and choices are greatly influenced not just by the 'facts' they are given, but by the way in which this information is presented to them, and so interpreted by them. This framing of the information can have a crucial influence in tipping the balance of decision. The doctor is wise to recognize that it is difficult, if not impossible to offer information that is value-free. It tends to be tinged with the doctor's own attitudes and values and may be slanted by the cues and hints which find their way into his exposition. Sometimes this is because of his previous observations of the outcomes, of which the patient has no comparable experience.

Interpreting statistical information

As the years pass, a doctor will accumulate a store of experience of outcomes, which moulds his views. Initially his databank is small, and he may be unduly biased by a single favourable or unfavourable outcome he has encountered. A firmer basis of judgement can often be derived from the published experience of others. But it is wise to guard against being professionally spellbound by marginal differences in statistical outcomes. For example, the observation that (say) a combination of radical surgery and aggressive chemotherapy results in a 2–3 per cent improvement in the five-year survival for a particular form of cancer, appears an unconvincing reason to recommend this form of treatment routinely to all-comers.

Even though statistical data about outcome may appear to be arithmetically objective, they are almost inevitably slanted by the way they are presented to the patient, especially one who may have limited ability to grasp the niceties of probability reasoning. For example, the risk that a pregnant epileptic woman taking two or more anticonvulsant drugs will have an infant with congenital abnormality is about 6 per cent, compared with a 'background' risk of around 2 per cent. If she is told 'your risk of an abnormal baby is three times greater than normal', this is likely to convey a very different message from an alternative interpretation of the same facts—'94 out of 100 babies will be normal and unaffected'.

Defensive information

Information offered to the patient may also be tainted by the fact that it is being given defensively to protect the doctor, rather than in a disinterested attempt to assist the patient's choice. The phraseology of contemporary consent for operation forms undoubtedly includes a major defensive component. The explanations which are certified as having been given to the patient are there to protect the doctor as much as, or perhaps even more than the patient.

Informed consent for operation is best assured with the additional help of a printed information sheet. This should cover the following points [73].

• the operation name, in lay terminology;

• nature of the problem being treated;

• nature of the proposed treatment;

• what the operation involves;

• other treatment options;

• potential complications (detail variable from patient to patient);

- success rate for the operation;
- what happens on admission;
- how you will feel afterwards;
- how long you are likely to be off work;
- special precautions, if any, needed post-operatively.

Such information packages covering more than a hundred general surgical operations are available on a computer disc.

The prescribing of drugs can also be accompanied by information that is given defensively. A body representing major drug manufacturers has suggested that patients should ask for, and doctors provide, much more detailed information about the individual drugs they receive. This appears laudable, but if the underlying motive is primarily to protect the doctor and/or the drug manufacturer, the type of information given and the way it is presented is likely to be biased.

Since January 1994, all new medicines are accompanied by patient information leaflets. Similar leaflets for established medicines are being phased in gradually. These leaflets tell patients how to use their medicines safely and effectively, and ask them to report undesirable effects to a doctor or pharmacist. About 10–20 per cent of all hospital in-patients experience some from of adverse reaction to drugs. These adverse reactions are of two types. Type A reactions are predictable, based on the pharmacological action of the drug, and are a consequence of level of dosage or reduced clearance. Type B reactions include hypersensitivity reactions. They are unpredictable (in the absence of a specific history), and are often severe or even fatal. The printed leaflets are only obligatory for medicines dispensed in an original pack, which does not apply to most hospital medicines.

A doctor may also be influenced in giving advice by personal considerations—the possibility of a surgical fee; the need to collect cases for a thesis or a research project; the fear of exposure to litigation.

Limiting information

Leaving aside these flaws, doctors are often very heavily influenced in the extent of the information they give to patients by a sincerely felt sense of duty to protect patients from needless anxiety. For example, few doctors would consider it professionally responsible to catalogue to each patient *all* the possible outcomes and complications of a particular operation or procedure (unless, perhaps, the patient was an American malpractice lawyer!) To do so could readily be adjudged cruelly alarmist and the worst sort of defensive medicine. A study of the effects of three different forms of pre-operative patient education in reducing anxiety showed that *detailed* information had the least favourable effect, and sometimes even increased anxiety.

Similarly, during the search for a diagnosis, a wise doctor will sometimes feel that he should set limits to the plethora of investigations to which the patient could be subjected. Ward [74] expressed the doctor's dilemma very clearly: 'Should I say to an anxious introspective patient with vague abdominal pain: "I am 95 per cent certain that you have no serious disease, but to remove the other 5 per cent of my lingering doubt that you might have cancer of the pancreas would require an invasive procedure with a 90 per cent diagnostic rate, but with an 0.5 per cent risk of serious complications, searching for a condition with only a one per cent five-year survival", or do I reassure them, and carry for them the burden of my slight uncertainty?'

Fully informed consent is not, as already indicated, a medico-legal requirement in Britain, and in any strict sense it is often an unattainable ideal. At a practical level, the aim should be to try to provide information which is:

(1) adequate for making well-founded decisions;

(2) not consciously biased;

(3) not unnecessarily alarming.

The learner, striving to improve his skills in this important part of the consultation, will often find it better to be guided as much by what the patient wants to know as by what the doctor thinks he should be told. The sort of helpful questions which might be asked are: 'Do you understand what needs to be done?' 'Is there anything more I can tell you?', 'Do you want to ask me any questions about that?', or 'Can I tell you anything more to help you decide?' The possibly relatively limited information that the patient actively seeks and the clarifications he is then offered may be much more helpful to him than a larger volume of gratuitous and perhaps indigestible detail.

RECOGNIZING DIFFERENT SCALES OF VALUES

In the language of decision theory, a rational choice is one that maximizes expected utility (or benefit). But this neat axiom masks the subjective nature of the value scales on which the assessment of benefit rests.

There is clear evidence that patients' and doctors' (or nurses') value scales are likely to diverge in several areas of medical decision-making. For example, during cancer chemotherapy, when toxic multiple-drug treatment is under consideration, the average patient is willing to opt for more unpleasant therapy, with smaller chances of cure or even relief, than the average doctor or nurse feels it is right to inflict on a patient [75].

Again, in the management of extremely premature infants in intensive care, mothers are more likely than nursing or medical staff to want to struggle to keep the infant alive however serious the risks of long-term handicap. Further, in evaluating those risks, nursing staff attach more importance to intact intellectual function (as against physical wholeness) than do mothers [76]. In both instances, it seems that clinging to life itself is more important for the patient than the relativities of quality of life, to which the professional staff attach greater value.

To take another example, this time of differing cultural values, P.R.M. found while practising obstetrics in the Sultanate of Oman, that most traditional Arab women are very reluctant to undergo Caesarean section for the sake of the baby. They prefer to keep the uterus intact for future child-bearing, though risking the loss of one child, rather than incurring an increased maternal risk in the current and every future pregnancy. And who could say that, in the setting of their lives, they are wrong!

Even within the same culture, patients in different circumstances are liable to adopt differing value scales. For example, when a decision has to be made about continuing a pregnancy in which there is a possible risk of fetal handicap (say following an acute viral infection in early pregnancy) differing views and values are likely to be held by:

- mothers of several healthy children;
- women whose pregnancy was preceded by long years of infertility;
- mothers who already have a handicapped child;
- mothers from countries where no support services for the handicapped exist.

Given, then, such differing value scales, valid for particular patients with their own circumstances, attitudes, and beliefs, great caution is advisable before dismissing a patient's choices as 'irrational' and therefore invalid. Some decision-making, however, does spring from irrational thinking. The patient may be swayed by irrational fear, of anaesthesia for example, or of contracting AIDS. Short-term benefit or pleasure may blind the patient to the delayed costs, as the behaviour of smokers, drinkers, and sunbathers demonstrates. Irrational convictions of invulnerability to modest risks are also common, especially among adolescents (seen, for example in the failure to use seat belts, crash helmets, or contraceptives).

Shared decisions

Often after open discussion the view of the doctor and the patient coincide, or at least can be reconciled in a mutually satisfactory way. The concept of a 'shared decision' provides a formula for compromise between the apparently irreconcilable notions of patient autonomy and of professional authority.

But because of different values, goals, and appreciation of risks and benefits, the patient and the doctor may sometimes come to different conclusions. The doctor is then faced with a dilemma between respect for the patient's autonomy, and a wish to protect the patient from choices which the doctor sincerely believes are harmful. Sometimes the difference of view is concerned with what is right or wrong in a moral sense.

Decision by proxy

Some patients, as we have seen, virtually hand over the responsibility for decisions: 'Well, you are the doctor. I will go along with whatever you advise.' This is perhaps the simplest example of decision by proxy. The doctor in effect decides for the patient, but with his expressed consent. In other proxy decisions a protective or paternalistic doctor may take it upon himself to make the decision (p. 118). But the situation becomes more complex ethically when a third party is involved and the decision has to be reached by a parent or relative, usually in close consultation with the doctor. The issue might be:

- deciding about the continuance of termination of pregnancy where there is fetal abnormality;

- deciding how vigorously to support the life of a newborn infant weighing only 750g, or of a seriously brain-damaged accident victim;

- deciding about the treatment of a demented elderly relative.

In extreme instances, a doctor or even a fourth party (such as a social work department), feeling that a child-patient's true interests are not being protected, may seek to make the child a ward of court. The power of decision is then taken out of the hands of individuals, and rests with the court.

THE DOCTOR'S GUIDANCE: THE EXPOSITION

At the point in the interview when the doctor is expected to give his opinion on the case, he must be ready to present the options and spell out clearly the reasons for his conclusions. The areas to be covered include the diagnosis and the prognosis; what needs to be done, or sometimes what little can be done; any medication to be prescribed, or any other specific treatment; and what action the patient should take [7]. Unhappily a survey by the Consumers Association among hospital out-patients showed that one in five leave the consulting room without understanding what is wrong with them, or knowing what the treatment will be (*Which* February 1991). A quarter of out-patients did not get *any* information on their condition from the consultant unless they asked for it.

There is good evidence that, with better interviewing, patients hear and hearken to the doctor's advice better [77,78]. Besides

promoting greater compliance, good communication is also likely
to reduce the need to prescribe drugs at all.

Practical considerations

If the exposition is to achieve its purpose, the doctor needs to
be properly prepared. In the first place, he should have brought
together the information on which his recommendations will be
based. When the interview follows various investigations and tests,
the doctor must ensure that he has the laboratory, X-ray, and
similar reports to hand. The efficiency of the filing and reception
staff in the case of an out-patient, or of the house officer in the case
of an in-patient, is vital in bringing together all the reports in good
time. It is most unsatisfactory if the doctor's recommendations are
qualified with all sorts of ifs and buts because information that
should have been available is not to hand. No amount of empathy
can compensate for absence of facts!

It is also vital that the doctor knows what the patient has already
been told, particularly in hospital, where different medical and
nursing staff may have given the patient information. Details of
this should always be carefully recorded in the case folder (p. 127).
Without the continuity that this written information promotes, the
patient is at risk of being given conflicting opinions and statements,
so that at the end of the day he may have a rather confused picture
of his illness and the proposed plan of management.

It is a wise precaution to have as much information as possible
regarding previous therapy. Nothing is more destructive of the
patient's confidence than an exchange such as:

'Now I'm going to prescribe for you some . . . which should quickly
relieve your . . .'

'But doctor, I was given that last year at the clinic, and it didn't
help. In fact, it made things worse!'

In addition to availability of information, a further element
contributes greatly to the patient's understanding of his condition.
This is the doctor's skill in choosing vocabulary suitable to the
patient. The form of words and choice of terms will differ from
one patient to another; it will be influenced by education, cultural
and occupational background, and other factors. Terms the doctor

may regard as 'innocent' and reassuring may readily create serious anxiety. For example, if a woman with a cervical erosion is told that she has 'just a small ulcer on the neck of the womb', she may infer the presence of serious disease, imminently or actually malignant, and be too alarmed to try to clarify what the doctor's words really mean. The middle-aged man with a sore back who is X-rayed and then reassured that it 'just shows some early arthritis in the spine', may associate the term arthritis with severe manifestations of advanced rheumatoid arthritis observed in a relative or acquaintance, and be convinced that he faces a future of crippling disability.

Therefore, it is often helpful not only to ask 'Do you understand that?' but also to invite the patient to say what *he* understands a particular diagnostic term of mean. Only by clarifying in this way can one be sure that the patient has a clear and correct idea of the nature of his illness.

Deferring the exposition

Sometimes at the end of a first interview, the doctor may wish (for a variety of reasons) to defer any exposition to a later occasion. He may feel unready to commit himself to a diagnosis, or a line of therapy until he has received the results of tests; he may wish to stall the patient's apparent expectation of medication; he may feel he needs to buy time to reflect on the case, and to get more information at a further interview. In these circumstances, the doctor should not hesitate to withhold his conclusions until a subsequent occasion.

He should also avoid dishing out a prescription that is not clinically necessary because he is unsure what else to do; because he is weary or short of time; because he wishes to pre-empt an argument; because he wishes to demonstrate concern; or because he can see no other neat way of bringing the interview to a conclusion [79].

COUNSELLING

When patients need help to resolve or, at least, reduce those sources of stress in their lives which are making them feel unwell, some form of counselling is usually the most effective therapeutic approach. The doctor who seeks to develop counselling skills must first recognize clearly the radical change in roles from those which tend to prevail in acute illness, especially in hospital. In the crisis of acute illness, a doctor is expected to demonstrate competence with authority, and to act decisively. But when offering counselling, he needs to adopt a quite different role, and deploy skilfully sapiential, moral, and charismatic qualities, which facilitate the functions of a counsellor. These include.

- Listening: evoking reactions and feelings.

- Providing information.

- Avoiding value laden opinions.

- Helping to define options and the consequences of choices.

- Providing continuing support.

The patient, who in acute illness is by and large exempted from normal obligations, and exonerated from any feeling of responsibility for his condition, has during counselling to face the challenge

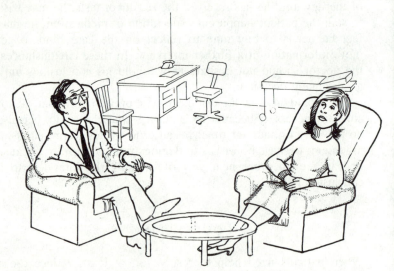

Fig. 10.1 An informal relaxed setting is appropriate for counselling

of decisions and choices which may involve fundamental changes in attitudes or behaviour. The dynamic for these changes can only come from within the patient himself. To identify the problems and the options for change, insight has to develop; to understand their implications and to assess their likely consequences, the patient's capacity for decision-making has to be mobilized; to maintain new directions, the patient's motivation has to be sustained. For the patient, reaching decisions may well be something hitherto ignored or avoided. A primary objective of counselling is to kindle in the patient a greater sense of purpose and volition.

A suitable ambience for non-directive dialogue of this nature is illustrated in Fig. 10.1.

AIDS TO RETAINING INFORMATION

Even when the utmost care is taken to explain matters clearly to the patient, subsequent enquiry often shows that the patient's recollection of what he has been told is incorrect or incomplete. This is not surprising when one considers how 'keyed up' the patient may have been at the time. Sometimes, the patient forgets to ask a question that has been pushed to the back of his mind by anxiety during the interview. On other occasions, he may have wanted to ask additional questions about matters of detail, but have felt he should not take up more of the doctor's time.

Particularly at the point when a patient is being discharged from hospital, there is almost inevitably a break in communication. There is often regrettable delay in writing to the family doctor. A telephone call may be forgotten. At the time of discharge, no doctor may be available to speak to the patient.

It can be very helpful, therefore, if each in-patient is given an information card [80,81] on leaving hospital, which provides guidance both for himself and for the family doctor. Out-patient consultations and in-patient interviews can be recorded on tape, so that the patient can digest the information further at home, and be reminded of important detail. This is particularly helpful for patients with cancer [82].

Written communication

THE USE OF THE CASE RECORD

While this book is primarily concerned with direct person-to-person communication, particularly in its affective aspects, something needs to be said about the written material relating to patients–the case records, letters, and so on–and the way in which these ought to complement and promote good interpersonal communication. If talking with the patient is to include the patient's feelings and concerns, this needs to be reflected in the written observations relating to the patient's care.

Clinical case records, of course, serve many functions: recording the history, clinical findings and investigation results, the details of treatment and the progress notes, as well as bringing together the correspondence between doctors. It can be useful for a student to study a few old case records carefully, and to try to trace the course of events—what was actually happening to the patient day-by-day during the course of the illness. Quite apart from problems of legibility, confusing abbreviations, undated entries, and so forth, and difficulties in piecing together the results of investigations, it is not easy to trace a coherent day-to-day account of the progress of the illness, and the patient's feelings and concerns do not usually attain even a passing mention. Sometimes there may be a brief initial comment, such as 'a pleasant, helpful, well-groomed lady', or perhaps 'a thin, anxious man, full of questions'. This may be all that is said in the whole record about the patient as a person, and such patronizing clichés betray more about the doctor who wrote them than they reveal about the patient!

Since 1 November 1991, patients have had a new right of access to all of their personal health records written after the same date, both in the National Health Service and in the private sector. This includes correspondence as well as clinical notes. The Medical

Defence Union has advised doctors not to write 'witty, derogatory, or even frankly offensive comments in the notes'. This new law is likely to improve the quality of the records, and should promote greater trust between patients and their doctors, though it might on occasion inhibit the expression of honest opinion from doctor to doctor [83].

It has to be acknowledged that the nursing Kardex record frequently provides a more comprehensible narrative than medical case records, and, more importantly, it often takes greater account of the affective aspects of illness, of how the patient is feeling. The differences between nursing and medical records are no accident, nor are they a consequence of the superior literary skills of nurses! These routine written reports on the progress of each patient, drafted by the nurse in charge, are the formal medium for communication of information whenever a new shift of nursing staff comes on duty. They are a necessary consequence of the pattern of nurse staffing, with its regularly defined hours of duty.

In contrast, resident medical staff have, in past years, remained on duty or on call for long and often indefinite periods of time, with no regular formal handover to another person or team. Information about patients was then provided verbally through the almost continuous availability of the resident house officer in person, so that there was less evident need for a comprehensive sequence of written observations in the case records.

Over the years, the pattern of medical junior hospital staffing has changed, and now regular rotas are worked in most instances, inevitably with a great deal of deputizing and transfer of clinical responsibility. Similarly, in general practice, doctors group together to share a duty roster during out-of-office hours, and the use of deputizing services is commonplace. But the pattern of medical record-keeping has not yet evolved in pace with these changes, and the need to ensure more systematic, complete transfer of information when a different individual or medical team takes over duty has still to be fully recognized.

Whatever system of recording is employed, it is important that the patient's affective concerns are identified, recorded, regularly updated, and kept under review. If this is done, any doctor who is on duty, and who may be dealing with the patient for the first time whether in hospital or in a group practice, is aware of what has been going on in the patient's mind and of his reactions to his illness. With this important background information, the doctor can 'tune in' to the patient much more effectively, and not feel a stranger. Similarly, a careful record needs to be made of what the patient is told, so that he does not receive dissonant or contradictory messages from different sources. This information should also be included in the letters interchanged between family and hospital doctors.

WRITTEN HANDOUTS AND INFORMATION BOOKLETS

It can often be helpful to make use of written leaflets or audiotapes to provide patients with supplementary information on a number of topics, particularly explanation and guidance regarding treatment. Some of these materials have already been referred to (pp. 116, 125). In my own clinical field, for example, handouts have been a regular part of antenatal care and preparation for parenthood for many years, but they are of value in many other situations. At the time of routine surgery, patients can be given a leaflet briefly describing their operation, with an account of what the operation implies, the course of post-operative recovery, return to normal activity, and so on (see p 116). Other varied examples of written material of this sort include dietary sheets, contraceptive advice, pamphlets about stoma care, information about male and female sterilization, recovery after a heart attack, and briefing notes for sex therapy. A helpful leaflet for parents who have just experienced the loss of a baby is available [55]. Patients who wish to know and understand more about their illness generally can be referred to books or booklets such as those published by the British Medical Association or by many patient self-help associations [39,40]. This type of information is especially important in chronic conditions such as diabetes mellitus, arthritis, colitis, whose management calls for changes in the patient's lifestyle and habits. A research study of patients' views on the information they would like to be given about prescribed drugs [84] showed that patients regarded the following details as particularly important:

• When and how to take the medicines.

• Unwanted (side) effects and what to do about them.

- Precautions (such as effects on driving).

- Interactions with alcohol or other drugs.

- The name of the medicine.

- The purposes of the drug treatment.

- What to do if a dose is missed.

Such detail is unlikely to be remembered accurately unless it is written down.

PATIENT RECORDINGS

Just as written materials can improve the quality of the information conveyed from doctor to patient, so the same is true in the reverse direction. Particularly when patients' symptoms are recurrent, chronic, or possibly cyclical, a diary of events, kept by the patient, can often help to elucidate the diagnosis. Menstrual and premenstrual calendars, diaries recording headaches, pelvic pains, skin eruptions, mood scores, or asthmatic attacks are examples. Diabetic and similar diaries are also invaluable in monitoring the response to drug therapy, and in evaluating the side-effects of drugs.

The ultimate written communication from patient to doctor is a 'living will'. This is an expression of the patient's wishes in the event of being overtaken by sudden illness during which meaningful communication is impractical, and from which worthwhile recovery is unlikely. It rests on an assumption that a change of mind could not have occurred.

12 Communication in the setting of primary care

A.N.M. HEWITT

The doctor–patient relationship is the cornerstone of general practice, and places great influence in the practitioner's hands. Most patient care starts in general practice, and most long-term care occurs in the community. Most patients have a general practitioner, who maintains a unique record of their medical history from cradle to grave. Having a long-term knowledge of and relationship with patients, their families and friends, within a social setting, gives a special insight into patients' problems. The doctor–patient relationship rests on good communication—the ability of practitioners to talk and listen to their patients and to appreciate their individual problems. The medical, social, and psychological setting is of paramount importance in understanding the patient as a whole person, and not just as a disease or a condition.

In general practice, the doctor does not control the agenda. The patient makes the appointment and presents the problem, sometimes with limited ability to describe or define the complaint. The doctor has no foreknowledge of what the problem might be, or which organ(s) might be affected. Patients are free to decide what to do with the advice or prescription offered, and if they are not satisfied they can get another partner to see them, or move to another practice for a new opinion. The idea that patients humbly present their problems and then the general practitioner makes sense of it all and dispenses paternalistic wisdom, is remote from reality. The doctor must be open and listen to the patient. He has to give time and space to discuss the problem(s). The great majority of diagnoses can be made from the history alone. About 5 per cent of diagnoses can be clinched by adding the examination, and only 1–2 per cent need the aid of investigations. It is clear from research findings that the only tool of real importance is the doctor's ability to listen, and while listening to reflect upon what the patient is saying.

A general practitioner's records cover both practice and hospital contacts, and often contain sensitive personal information. While hospital letters summarize important factual information about episodes of illness and diagnoses, the reactions of patients to these events, and their efforts to come to terms with the stresses of their lives are no less important. It is in this area that primary care comes into its own. Detailed knowledge of patients and their families, with a comprehensive record of medical problems garnered over a period of time, provides a longitudinal view of health problems which can make general practice a most satisfying career.

TIMING

The opportunities for repeated contacts allow the tempo of communication to be varied in a much more flexible manner than is generally possible in hospital practice. It is useful and proper in general practice sometimes to talk about things that have little to do with the reason for the consultation. It is normal to adopt an ordinary conversational manner, as one might do with intimates at home. Patients appreciate the relaxed individual atmosphere. Many of us are very good at chatting with friends and putting them at ease, but unfortunately medical education can suppress these skills, making the doctor appear professionally distant. In general practice these skills are important tools.

During repeated contacts, practitioners observe gradual changes in patients' attitudes, feelings, and motivation. In some cases this can be likened to a maturing or ripening process, while in others there is a sense of decline, or missed opportunity. By deliberately extending periods of follow-up, more intimate knowledge of the person is acquired, and their trust is deepened.

Against this background, the practitioner can use his skill and experience to judge the best time for interventions or initiatives, waiting till the tide is favourable for change, when success is more likely.

DIAGNOSIS; 'GETTING A NOSE FOR IT'

There is a great satisfaction in making a diagnosis, especially of a condition which is rare, or which presents in an unusual manner.

The doctor can expect the compliments of colleagues as well as the gratitude of the patient. Untangling the slender strands of important information from the trivia is very satisfying, and not dissimilar to a detective story.

Some doctors in all specialities gain admiration from their fellows, most obviously for their diagnostic skill, their facility for communicating with patients, and for the degree of empathy they demonstrate. Underlying these capabilities is an ill-defined but quite distinct entity, related to the acumen of the doctor, which I shall call 'getting a nose for it'.

An expert wine taster can identify a wine and its characteristics—not only the type of grape and the year of harvesting, but even the particular vineyard from which it came. The grand master's special skill is a literal example of 'getting a nose for it'. However, this sort of complex skill can be demonstrated in many areas of professional and personal life. It involves a synthesis of experience and knowledge of a subject, and an alert observation, coupled with ability to use ideas both from within and outwith the profession. These abilities have been described by Schön as 'knowing an action' and 'reflection in action'. [129].

Knowing an action is something we all do regularly; we can recognize a condition without having to put all the bits and pieces of information together and then formally adding them up to make a diagnosis. It is similar to seeing a familiar face, and knowing who the person is without having to analyse all their particular features.

Reflecting in action is more complex. We use this skill when we come up against a problem for which there is no obvious answer. While trying to find a solution, we begin to call on knowledge and skills from outside our normal range, gleaned possibly from general reading, experience of life, or from other professional disciplines. This ability allows us to handle problems which we have not come across before, and did not know we could resolve.

It has been said (ironically) that in general practice one can regularly make a diagnosis before the patient has settled in the seat, write a prescription, and have the patient out of the surgery within 90 seconds! This may be true when there is some simple physical diagnosis, but it is nonsense in regard to the problems commonly presented in the surgery, more than half of which have a primarily psychological component. One can literally 'get a nose for' diabetes or for an anaerobic wound infection quite easily, but what about situations which are less clear-cut, involving psychological and emotional upset, such as various forms of abuse. Even when the doctor feels that all is not right, how does he or she begin to talk about what the 'nose' suspects? How are such difficult areas approached?

Abuse

The term 'abuse' has become a common contemporary label for a variety of unacceptable forms of behaviour. All doctors have come across the abuse of alcohol and other drugs. Many doctors will have experience of patients who have themselves been subjected to physical or sexual abuse, often as children. Because these behaviours attract general disapprobation, they are kept as dark secrets.

Sometimes patients are encountered who present their problems in such a manner that, at the end of the consultation, the doctor is left totally confused. These situations are likely to arise when the patient has emotional problems which they find it difficult to express or to cope with. Such problems may stem from some form of abuse.

Occasional patients appear to have a chaotic, disorganized, and dysfunctional lifestyle, in a social setting that the doctor does not understand. Travellers, for example, may seem to a settled householder to have a very odd way of life, but one which is perfectly 'normal' for them. However, there are situations that appear unequivocally dysfunctional. Patients, for example, who repeatedly take overdoses are found, in a significant proportion of cases, to have suffered abuse within the family. Awareness of this possibility has to be linked with sensitive timing—knowing when to enquire more deeply and how to pose the questions appropriately.

The practitioner must often adopt an indirect approach, at a pace which eases the patient forward, but avoiding abrupt confrontation which might well cause the patient to back off. Offering empathy and musing aloud may be helpful. 'To keep taking overdoses seems to me a strange thing to do. I wonder if you aren't very unhappy at times.' 'From my experience there is often a reason—something that happened to you in the past, leaving you feeling angry or depressed.' By this sort of exploration the practitioner can try to disarm the patient's defences, and so the real problems which underlie the dysfunctional behaviour can be brought to light.

Abused children almost always present themselves in some way, but rarely is the problem overt. It is important to use the 'nose' before too much damage is done. Contacts with the family, especially in the home, enable the practitioner to extend knowledge and understanding of the social environment. Often the relatives and friends of the family will be known, and information through them can be very helpful. Odd remarks may come from third parties such as aunts or uncles—'You know John? He really is getting out of hand. He used to be the bright one of the family.' Such information should be noted, at least in the doctor's memory. The 'nose' suggests something may be wrong, and the excuse that John is just a rebellious teenager may not provide the full answer.

To broach the topic, when John's mother next appears, the doctor could engineer an innocent sounding question: 'How are the family?' 'How old is John now? He must be growing up?' Because of the trusting relationship built up over time, and the knowledge that confidentiality will be observed, the mother may then speak frankly, but may not fully understand the situation. She also may think it is all just teenage rebellion. The practitioner must move on 'Have you thought what might be the problem?' 'Do you think it could be something more serious?' Slowly the doctor prods, and offers suggestions. There comes a point where the mother will either deny vehemently any major problem, or signal readiness for a serious discussion. 'Could John be taking drugs?' 'Has he been bullied at school?' 'Has he been abused in the home in the past or present?' Responsibility for handling this sort of important information can be frightening, especially when it is given in confidence by a third party

Reflection

There are other reasons why a doctor may sometimes feel totally nonplussed at the end of a consultation. It may be that the doctor has failed to ask the right questions or failed to listen carefully; the reflective mode has been switched off. Dysfunctional consultations may be related also to the patient's inner confusion, due to experiencing deep-seated unease or unhappiness which consciously they do not wish to acknowledge, let alone to understand. In this situation general practitioners are in the fortunate situation of knowing that the patient is likely to return in the not too distant future. They have an opportunity to reflect after the consultation, to note this in the record, and to use their 'nose'. The next time that patient appears, the doctor can pick up the threads, comment on the previous unsatisfactory consultation, and seek to explore the patient's real problems.

Frequent consultations

All general practitioners have patients who consult at least once a week. It is not unknown for some patients to consult over 100 times in a year! Because of the deluge of visits, the consultation is often dealt with as quickly and superficially as possible, with minimal effort. But the patient is likely to have a problem—a hidden agenda. Practitioners may fear that tackling this may open a 'can of worms', and throw up unsurmountable problems. But as the ability to develop 'a nose for it' grows, so too will the doctor's confidence in seeking solutions. Michael Balint in the 1950s led groups of practitioners who discussed their problem cases with each other over a period of time. Even though some problems were insoluble, the participants learnt to understand more of patients' motivation, and were able to help patients gain insight and come to terms with their problems.

COMMUNICATION WITHIN THE EXTENDED FAMILY OF CARERS

The nuclear family, mother, father, and children, exists in some form for most patients at some time in their lives. But children leave home; grandparents come to stay. Parents eventually may need care in a nursing home. A solitary old man may stay stubbornly in his own house, looked after by neighbours, social workers, and other carers. The concept of an extended family takes on added dimensions, where ethical and communication problems arise. Further issues of confidentiality pose practical questions of who to tell and how much to tell.

While it is possible to play it by ear, hoping to remain sufficiently alert to avoid inevitable pitfalls, some guidelines for action are necessary, avoiding rigid rules. The patient is regarded as having an overriding right to confidential access to information concerning themselves, while relatives, even the spouse, have no right to know. Yet this principle is not as absolute as it might be in the case of (say) a priest. We frequently share information with other health professionals—doctors, nurses, physiotherapists, etc. We also share information within the family when, for example, parents are informed of a child's problems. We readily justify this behaviour as something necessary for the patient's treatment. The parent has responsibility for the child, so passing on information directly helps care.

However, in primary care the concept of family is extended far beyond this narrow confine. It is impossible to practise in the community and maintain high standards of care without the involvement of an extended family of carers.

The legal situation of minors has become less clear-cut in recent times. Traditionally, the parent is responsible for the child up to the age of 16 years, and the child's right to confidentiality can be breached if it is in the interest of their health. Newer ethical concepts have affected this position, and now children have a claim to confidentiality at any age provided that they can understand what is being said to them, and the implications of any decisions taken. The thrust is to make a judgement about each patient on the basis of an individual assessment, taking all factors into account.

The most obvious example of this change is the 13-year-old girl coming to the general practitioner by herself and asking for the contraceptive pill. Should she be seen alone? Should she be prescribed the pill at all, when it is illegal to have intercourse under the age of sixteen? This particular dilemma has been discussed at length, and a measure of consensus prevails. She should be given the pill if she needs it, but should be advised to tell her parents herself. The general practitioner should counsel her carefully. However, the guidelines in other situations are not as clearly spelled out.

There is general agreement that communication with other health professionals is essential to deliver good care, through a network of shared information. But in the home, while the district nurse tends to nursing needs, and the practitioner to medical needs, many other people may be involved in care.

Consider a common situation where an old person is living at home. The house is too big for the old man, he does not heat it properly, and the gas cooker is ancient. The son and daughter live in a town about 30 miles away, and visit weekly. The district nurse visits regularly, as the old man has leg ulcers. The home help comes daily to make sure that there is at least one decent meal cooked each day, and she does the washing, and makes sure the shopping is done. The practitioner attends fairly regularly, endeavouring to control congestive cardiac failure, despite poor drug compliance. The next door neighbour pops in every morning to check all is well, and every evening to make a cup of tea, and check that the old man is settled for the night. The social services have given him an alarm, in case he falls and needs to summon help. Finally, the priest calls occasionally as the patient can no longer get to church.

In this common scenario, the doctor and nurse are the people with responsibility for seeing that each person involved has some information, because all are essential in sustaining the old person in his own home. Together, they form a complex network of interdependent support, in which everyone's role is important. The persons involved and their roles could be changed and extended in different scenarios. The general practitioner must co-ordinate the flow of information so that all involved remain confident and concerned in the task of caring.

There may also be social problems of significance. The patient has been depressed with suicidal thoughts, and in the past has abused alcohol. His family dislike him because he abused their mother when they were young, and was uncaring towards them. Do the nurse, the home help, or the neighbour need to know the origins of his depression? This is where the problems of passing confidential information really begin. The nurse and doctor customarily share a great deal of information within a concept of confidentiality that is equally understood. The good district nurse will weave topics and ideas into her everyday conversation, and the patient, reacting to these, provides a flow of information that brings better understanding of his problems, and better care. But what about the cheerful supportive home help? Would her enthusiasm be diminished if she knew what the old man had been like in earlier life? Her judgement that 'the old man is lovely with a great sense of humour' could be considerably altered if she knew the background. At present, her contact buoys up the old man, who really looks forward to her daily visits. However, it could be helpful if the home help knew of the alcohol problem, since she does the shopping and clears up round the house. She would be one of the first to know if the old man's intermittent bouts of confusion were caused by alcohol.

The good neighbour, like the home help. thinks the old man is lovely. 'Isn't it a pity that the family visit only once a week, and then only for half an hour!' Does she need to know that the family are merely fulfilling a duty and have no great love for their father? Would this help her understanding, or just create trouble?

Finally, what do the children need to know of the diagnosis and prognosis? Should they just be told the bare facts, or should the message be slanted to try and get them to be more involved? Since each situation is unique, judgements have to be based on an individual assessment. The complex web of interaction needs to be teased out so that each carer receives appropriate information to fulfil their role constructively. Again, listening to the carers' questions and asking a few simple questions of them may be all that is needed. 'Are you getting on OK?' 'Do you need any help?' 'Are there any problems?' 'Do you need to know anything else?'

The non-medical carers are often concerned that they do the right things, and they need the doctor's support. The home help may simply report, if given the opportunity, that there are lots of empty bottles. The next door neighbour, if simply told that there are family stresses, will then have sufficient insight into the family's detached behaviour. However, it is important that the general practitioner does not lose sight of the limits of confidentiality. For instance, a prying neighbour may have to be told bluntly that they are fishing for information to which they have no right. The doctor must always remain the patient's advocate and friend.

SHARING INFORMATION IN TERMINAL ILLNESS

A general practitioner is sometimes confronted by the spouse or children of a terminally ill patient. While the patient may be still in the dark, they have learnt the diagnosis from the staff in hospital. Because their own fears make them perceive the information as dreadful, the family wishes with the best of intentions to protect the dying person, and so they beg the doctor not to tell the patient the truth.

But how can the primary care team meet the patient's needs for care and support while evading the most important issue? If this situation develops, it blights relationships and destroys any real chance of meaningful communication. This in turn diminishes the quality of the care that can be given. The members of the primary care team have to take the family into their confidence and discuss their fears and concerns. Why should the patient be kept in ignorance? What do they fear would happen if he learnt the truth? The family need open opportunities to express their apprehensions. Do they properly understand the diagnosis and its implications? Possibly the feared word 'cancer' is all that they have picked up, and communication to support the family may be just as important as direct support for the patient.

Most doctors feel that patients should know their diagnosis, and families can often be persuaded to abandon their veto. This creates an opportunity to tackle real issues and to give genuine support to all involved as the illness progresses. The general practitioner can broach questions that may be in the patient's mind, which can be picked up at will. In this way the patient can be helped to confront and deal with his or her own fears and is no longer at the receiving end of everyone else's anxieties.

PROTECTION IN DEMENTIA

When an old person suffers from dementia, their autonomy is reduced as their wishes cannot be consulted fully, and their capacity to give or withhold consent is weakened because of their mental condition. While such a person is living at home, they may live in difficult circumstances, but they do maintain some autonomy. If they enter a residential home, their physical care may well be of a higher standard, but inevitably their autonomy is reduced. The routines of a residential home, like that of a hospital, have to be maintained for everyone's good. The staff are not only carers, but they often assume family roles as they help the patient through everyday situations. Unlike most staff in hospital, they have continuing contact with the patient in what has now become

the patient's home. Their role as carers can become confused with
that of friend and confidant, with much of the influence that a
family member might have. The genetic family is relieved of the
task of caring, but may well retain a legal responsibility for the
patient's money and property.

In such situations the patient's autonomy, privacy, and right to
confidentiality can be in jeopardy, and the general practitioner can
be in a difficult situation. He must keep the patient's interests
uppermost, even though it is not always clear where those interests
lie. If, to take the simplest example, a fracas occurs when a helper
is trying to change the clothing or bathe the patient, can the doctor
turn a blind eye to the rumpus, confident that the yelling and
shouting is just because the elderly patient is having something
done to them for their own good? Does the patient have the
right to object, despite their dementia, or have they surrendered
that right?

The general practitioner's role is to monitor the patient's care
and treatment objectively, and to remain the patient's advocate
and the defender of their interests generally.

CONFIDENTIALITY AND PARTNERS

When the general practitioner is looking after a man and a woman
living together, questions of confidentiality arise. Does one partner
have any right to know about the other's health problems? If the
unmarried couple have been living together for some time, and
especially if they are looking after their own children, there may
be little problem. There is an assumption that this is a form of
marriage, and should be so treated. But what is reasonable period
of cohabitation before the doctor can presume a form of marriage?
When do they stop being just lovers and become a 'married
couple' with the expectation that confidences can be shared? It
may create hostility to jump in and enquire about the status of
the relationship directly—'By the way, are you two together for
keeps, or just lovers passing in the night?' The situation can be less
easy with a homosexual couple, who could be in the equivalent of
a marriage, sharing everything including the mortgage, or they may
be just good friends. The practitioner, too, might find difficulty in
understanding or accepting a homosexual relationship.

CONCLUSION

When communicating with their patients in the setting of primary care, doctors need to become aware of their own styles of consulting, and the way in which their own personalities, strengths, and weaknesses can affect their ability to help patients deal with problems.

'In general practice the patient can have any disease he likes, or none at all.' This quotation underlines the fact that patients are their own masters, and they are often on their own territory, or at least on the familiar ground of the practice surgery. Their symptoms will sometimes sound confusing, and they will be talking apparently about conditions that are not as described in medical textbooks. These circumstances can present a threat to the confidence of the less experienced doctor, who may feel the need to exercise his authority, to take control of the conversation, and to impose a diagnosis or solution. If this happens, the patient is liable to feel alienated, confidence will be lost, and care will be compromised. Benefit for the patient, as well as professional satisfaction for the doctor, is more likely to result from a patient-centred approach, where the patient's agenda remains uppermost.

13 Talking about babies

I.A.LAING

INTRODUCTION

There is a common misapprehension that neonatology is diminished as a specialty because infants cannot articulate, and therefore there is little need for good communication. On the contrary, the neonatologist is meeting the needs of a family, often at the most stressful time of young parents' lives. High expectations of a normal pregnancy and delivery, with a resultant delightful infant, are shattered when at (say) 24 weeks gestation a creature hardly recognizable as human emerges and is cocooned for weeks or months within the confines of a transparent plastic box in a strange intensive care unit. At no time can it be more important for a physician to impart information clearly, pitching the dialogue at a level appropriate for a single unsupported mother, a mutually supportive couple, or the entire family involved. This chapter first touches briefly on talking to infants themselves. Discussions with parents during the normal newborn examination are then described. Finally, we consider ways of communicating with families during the special stresses of neonatal intensive care, when hopes for a normal outcome are entangled with fears of death or major handicap.

TALKING TO BABIES

Gone are the days when new-born babies were regarded as almost insentient beings who could be wakened and heel-stabbed at will. Intubation, assisted ventilation, chest drains, and even major operations were in time past carried out without regard for the pain experienced by the child, who could do little to protest.

The newborn infant does feel pain [85] and has now been shown to have a worse clinical outcome if analgesia to block the stress response is inadequate [86,87]. Work is currently being undertaken to establish the influence of soothing words and pleasant social touch in rehabilitating the sick infant[88].

The infant can hear, and families should be encouraged to talk to their new baby. In the intensive care unit bonding is promoted by coaxing the closest family members to open incubator portholes and touch, stroke, and speak encouraging words to the infant. Some parents, matching the high technology of special care, will even persuade an older sibling of the baby to record fairy stories and nursery rhymes which can then be played back to the new-born, using small speakers inside the incubator.

But should the doctor talk to the new-born infant? There are three reasons why the answer is 'yes'. First, the new-born is soothed by the sound of the human voice, and during clinical examination more information becomes available; auscultation of the heart is more revealing, assessment of tone is more reliable, and palpation of the abdomen becomes easier. Second, the child's parents are more likely to have confidence in a clinician who is seen to talk to and care for the child as a dignified individual rather than as an object being inspected Third, the anxious novice doctor feels more at ease during his examination if it becomes fun, and the sense of confidence spreads to other members of the care-giving team and to the family. The early hours of a child's life remain locked in the parents' memory; they should be a special and a joyous time.

TALKING TO PARENTS

The perfect communicator is also the perfect listener. Parents can harbour anxieties that the compulsive talker will never recognize or even suspect. What is trivial to the clinician may be momentous to a father or mother—one mother whose child had just been put under a phototherapy light confided 'I feel as though my right arm has been cut off'. The sympathetic acceptance of irrational dread can be a vital prelude to conveying reassurance to parents. The most stressful circumstances in neonatal care involve life-threatening congenital abnormalities, perinatal asphyxia, extreme prematurity, and neonatal death.

Congenital abnormalities

Ultrasound scanning of the fetus has brought about a revolution in perinatal care, and parents can often be warned in advance about certain congenital abnormalities. In the case of defects which are incompatible with life, both father and mother will often have had the opportunity to begin the grieving process before the birth of the infant.

However, many congenital abnormalities are as yet undetectable by screening, and detailed scanning cannot be offered for all pregnancies. Unexpected defects are therefore still found at birth, and these must be described and explained with accuracy and sensitivity to the family. In the past there was a prevalent view that delay in explanation was desirable to allow time for parents to bond to the child before any bad news was communicated. A more enlightened view is that all delays increase parental anxieties and fuel distrust towards the professional care-givers. Early rapport and early information with assurance of support are preferable to letting the parents build a false joy today which will be cruelly shattered tomorrow.

All information shared needs to be founded on factual evidence. The senior paediatrician should assess what is known, what more can be discovered, and what is unpredictable. Some conditions look terrifying to parents but are eminently treatable, while others appear benign but are of disastrous consequence. Gastroschisis, a condition in which the intestines are extruded through a defect in the abdominal wall, is cosmetically one of the most appalling conditions that a parent may be confronted with. Yet with expert management in the early hours of life the defect can be repaired and the family can look forward to bringing up a child with a normal future. In contrast, incontinentia pigmenti presents like a linear nettle rash in a new-born infant and can be laughingly dismissed by the unwary. But within the first two years of life the associated microcephaly, seizures, and neuro-developmental delay are often apparent. To protect families from being given misinformation at an early stage, which then has to be corrected, staff at all levels need continuing education, and neonatal consultants have to find time to be involved in the personal delivery of care.

BREAKING BAD NEWS

How best should the doctor say to a couple 'Your child has Down's syndrome?' There is no universal answer, for much depends on the personalities of the communicator and the parents, the circumstances involved, and whether the parents already suspect that all is not well. In her book *Will, my son* [89], Sarah Boston recounts how she resented having been told the diagnosis when her child's father was not present. If the father is involved, whether married or not, it is important that the couple should be given the news together—the same information in the same language at the same time. The neonatologist will have considered the possibility that the diagnosis of Down's syndrome is wrong, including the rare circumstance of mosaicism, when the prognosis may be better. If, however, the child's appearance leaves little doubt, it is unwise to offer frightened parents the false hope that perhaps the chromosomal findings will turn out to be less serious than feared. It is much better to speak frankly 'I am sorry to tell you that your baby has Down's Syndrome, which means that he/she will present special difficulties for you over the coming months and years'.

Good practice involves ensuring that the people principally involved are present, and no one else—the mother, father, maybe a close family member, and the midwife/nurse who has developed a relationship with the mother during labour. Sometimes, the presence of a social worker, the general practitioner, or a medical or nursing student might be appropriate. The distressed couple could be helped by having their three-year-old daughter with them, strengthening their sense of family.

Doctors, finding such interviews stressful, are sometimes liable to take refuge in technical descriptions, but rather than retreating into an account of non-disjunction or Brushfield spots, it is better to attempt a basic explanation of what the child's future is likely to be. The support available within the community, including special education and physiotherapy, can be outlined. Often, it is most helpful to introduce the couple to another family who have a child with Down's syndrome. They can best empathize with them, and explain where they found solace, encouragement, and practical guidance when facing a similar turmoil in their lives.

Perinatal asphyxia

Few situations can be more terrifying for a mother than to deliver a baby and then find that the infant, blue and lifeless, has been pounced on by a paediatric team, who are devoting all their attention to resuscitation, seemingly heedless of the presence of the parents. For the senior house-officer in the neonatal unit many resuscitations are just routine, but for the scared parents, warning beforehand about likely procedures can be of great comfort. When an unpredicted emergency occurs, the resuscitator should find time for a few words with the parents 'I'm afraid your baby is having difficulty in starting to breathe and we are giving help with this. It will be a few more minutes before we know whether this is a serious problem, but I promise we will not hide anything from you.' Once the child has been stabilized, there is almost always time for the parents to greet their new infant for the first time, even though the baby may be flaccid and immobile on a portable ventilator, en route to the neonatal unit. Mother can still put her hand through the portholes of the transport incubator and stroke the forehead of her new offspring. The senior paediatrician present should assure the parents that the child is being taken to intensive care, will be stabilized on the equipment, and that further information will be given to the parents with all speed.

The principle that all information imparted should be soundly based on facts applies here very strongly. The wise clinician builds a prognosis based on the degree of hypoxic ischaemic encephalopathy, as measured by seizures, tone, and overall neurological activity, as well as insults to other organs. The messages to parents are not based simply on the condition of the child at the time of birth, but more especially on the evolution of the clinical picture as the hours and days go by. 'We are concerned that during the first six hours your baby has not yet started to breathe, and the ventilator has had to do all the work. This makes us very concerned about the possibility of damage to the brain. The coming hours will make the situation clearer, and we will talk about it again then.' Initially parents may feel stunned, or angry that something has 'gone wrong'. They must be assured that they will be afforded every opportunity to discuss the situation again and again. They must be left in no doubt that their opinions about future management are important, and that the care-givers will work with the parents as a team to try to provide the best outcome for the child, whatever that may be.

Extreme prematurity

Developments in obstetrics, midwifery, neonatal nursing, and paediatrics have resulted in extraordinary improvements in outcome for extremely preterm infants. Management of the infant born at 28 weeks has become routine in the intensive care units of the developed world, with the expectation of survival and normal development. For the child born at 24 weeks, however, this is far from the case. The parents face the possibility of early death, or a long arduous course probably involving prolonged assisted ventilation until survival is attained. The child's future may be marred by special needs including continued respiratory support and neuro-developmental disabilities. A balanced perspective has to be struck in the face of these uncertainties in the road ahead.

The first visit of parents to the neonatal intensive care unit is, for them, akin to stepping on to the flight deck of Concorde and being expected to understand the controls immediately. They come to meet their baby, but are faced with complex machines, whose sounding alarms are apparently being ignored by the staff. Their tiny infant is dwarfed by an oxygen monitor, a pulse oximeter, an endotracheal tube, two temperature probes, three intravenous infusions, an umbilical arterial catheter, and a napkin seemingly designed for quite a different species. For the staff, the challenge is to introduce the parents to the machinery, only so that they can then ignore it, and focus on their child. If a first name has been chosen by the parents, this should be used consistently.

All of us fear what we do not understand, and parents in this situation demonstrate this most clearly. Written information should be available for parents to take away so that they can study a basic explanation of neonatal intensive care in their own home. Some clinicians audiotape the interview with mother and father, so that this explanation of what is happening to their child and what the future holds can be re-played at will. Parents are encouraged to write down questions and bring them at their next visit. 'This sounds stupid but . . .?' is a common parental approach to some salient point which has been overlooked by the staff.

Senior staff cannot devote several hours per week discussing the anxieties of every parent, but those under most stress require repeated meetings, the content of which needs to be documented in the case record, so that other members of the unit will use the same language to convey consistent information. Although the standard of communication is often satisfactory during acute events, it may become woefully inadequate when a chronic phase of slow progress has been entered. The infant who has progressed from the ventilator but who needs to breathe an oxygen-enriched atmosphere for several months can impose untold frustration on parents whose lives are endlessly disrupted by travelling and visiting, irregular meals, and poor sleep patterns. Their need for regular support is easily overlooked.

Death

Neonatal death may occasionally occur suddenly and unexpectedly; the term infant delivered apparently free of congenital abnormalities may collapse and die in the first week of life due to hypoplasia of the left heart. More often, neonatal death is a predictable event involving inexorable deterioration, and parents may then begin the grieving process prior to the death of their baby. Although in both situations the needs of the infant and parents are paramount, the feelings of loss and sometimes guilt experienced by the staff are also very real.

Sensitive communication with the family will assist in creating a feeling of dignity around the time of the infant's death. Parents often prefer to share the intimacy of the event with just a small coterie of selected individuals. The senior paediatrician, the nurse who knows the family best, and perhaps one student may prove a suitable group, allowing necessary privacy for the family, but also an opportunity for less experienced staff to learn for the benefit of future families. Staff must be responsive to any clues when deciding the timing of actions and words. The young parents may never have seen a dead body before. They will insistently seek reassurance that their child is peaceful and undistressed, that every move is the right thing to do, and 'the best thing for baby'. They can be guided calmly, with empathy and support, through the last minutes of the child's life [90]. They should be given every opportunity to participate in holding, grooming, disconnecting monitors, dressing the baby, and then cuddling it after the consultant has removed the endotracheal tube. The parents may obtain solace from members of staff joining in the circle of baptism, or from talking about good times in the past or hopes for the future. It may seem macabre to involve an older sibling, but this is not so. The three-year-old elder sister may bring the family together, and will generally be unafraid to help, to comb the baby's hair, and to choose a doll for the baby to have in the coffin. Moments like these are precious, and likely to be indelible in the parents' memories. If the team can talk to all members of the family, listening, encouraging and providing guidance, but also giving them privacy as they wish, then much can be accomplished.

PROFESSIONAL SUPPORT

Doctors can often feel depressed, isolated, insecure, and physically and emotionally exhausted under the stressful circumstances of intensive care. They therefore need an effective organized system of professional support, encompassing all the health professionals involved. This is not easy to organize in an already overstretched service. The support function needs to be built into the regular working pattern of the unit—clinical rounds, case discussions, mortality reviews, etc. As the hours of duty worked by junior doctors are reduced, they are exposed to less pressure. The continuity of medical care can then only be delivered through the consultant, and it is entirely appropriate that this is so.

14 Talking to children

A.L. SPEIRS

Many doctors, other than paediatricians, have to deal with sick children. General practitioners, orthopaedic and ENT surgeons, eye and skin specialists all find that children make up a significant proportion of their patients. Therefore, most clinicians need to learn how to conduct a consultation with parent and child with consideration, care, and understanding. This is an essential requirement if the consultation is to achieve its objectives. Some doctors are regarded as naturally good with children, but through training, experience, and patience these skills can be developed and improved.

Paediatric patients encompass a wide span from the new-born to the adolescent. Parents range widely in social class, intelligence, and cultural background. The doctor therefore varies his approach, his questioning and his explanation accordingly. Indeed, this is one of the challenges and pleasures of working with children of different ages and backgrounds.

FEATURES AFFECTING THE SUCCESS OF THE INTERVIEW

Ideally, parents should be asked to prepare their child for a visit to a health centre or hospital, though probably few do so effectively. They should try to give a simple account of what is to happen: that the child is going to see a kind doctor who is going to try to help him. If possible, the child should be reassured that he is not going to be left behind in hospital, for though he may not show it, this notion can cause much anxiety. However, the vast majority of children are now treated as out-patients. It is very wrong at any time to reassure the child falsely simply to get him to come along.

On the child's arrival at the clinic, there should be a welcoming atmosphere and a cheerful receptionist; a waiting area used by children should provide facilities for play, and there should be an area for feeding and changing babies. In children's hospitals, the whole environment is geared for children, but general hospitals need to make more provision for the many children who attend them, and an effort should be made to separate children from adults not only in the wards but also in out-patients and casualty. Long waiting times are to be avoided, as young mothers usually have many domestic commitments and the children can get very restless and impatient.

A consulting room regularly used for children should be bright, with warm colours and cheerful murals, without overdoing the latter. A small chair and table with toys appropriate to a range of ages and both sexes can be available. Sometimes a doll's house or some picture books keep small children so happy that they do not want to leave. Children aged six or seven years upwards prefer a more formal approach and are quite happy to sit with mother. There should be no unpleasant instruments around other than those used in routine examination, such as a stethoscope, torch, or auriscope. Doctors rarely wear white coats nowadays and so avoid a 'clinical' atmosphere that might intimidate a child.

When mother and child are invited into the consulting room, the doctor should smile and welcome them by name, offer them a seat and introduce any other staff present. Communication is best when mother and doctor sit near each other without a large desk intervening. The doctor should have his desk on his right-hand side thus giving him easy access to the child who will be facing him and close to mother on his left side.

PRESENCE OF OTHERS IN THE ROOM

Privacy is important in all consultations and there is no reason for omitting this in the case of children. Unfortunately, in hospital it is not always possible to ensure complete privacy because of the presence of nurses, students, or others, but mothers will accept these circumstances provided they feel their child is going to be helped. If, at any time, the doctor considers privacy is essential (or if the mother requests it), he can ask the attendants to leave. Greater privacy usually prevails in general practice.

It is very useful to have a health visitor in the room, as she can provide the doctor with background information from her colleagues in the community and can in turn feed back useful information to them. After the interview, the mother should be given an opportunity to have a further informal chat in an adjacent room with the nurse or health visitor, so that anything she has not understood can be explained in simple terms. The nurse can speak with authority if she has been in the room during the consultation, and this avoids giving answers at variance with what the doctor has said. The health visitor can later pay a visit to the home if this is thought advisable.

THE HISTORY

Information from the mother

Obtaining information from the parent is a vital part of the consultation. The doctor should proceed slowly, feeling his way and gradually building up a picture of the child, his illness, and the family background. The real problem may be revealed only when a closer relationship has been established. Prying at an early stage can destroy an attempt to achieve good communication. In paediatric consultations, communication takes a triangular form, involving the doctor, the child, and the parent, each giving and receiving information, each observing and being observed. As the interview proceeds it is hoped that the mother will gain confidence in the doctor and will confide more, especially if the doctor is interested and relaxed and seems to have time to spend. If the child senses that his mother is more at ease he will respond similarly.

Junior doctors are trained in the early stages of their career to work through the history following a set format, but with experience, they learn to modify their interviewing technique (see p. 27). An unstructured approach is more natural, and effective, leaving the mother free to talk in her own fashion with only an occasional prompting or lead question being necessary. New angles will emerge that may need following through, but still the doctor must remember to return to the mainstream of the interview and not forget vital questions, for example about the perinatal period and the socio-economic background. During periods that are intensely emotional, it is appropriate to set aside note-taking and devote all attention to what the mother is saying. The notes can be completed after the mother has gone.

Although the *child* is the patient, the mother is a key person. Indeed, in infancy particularly, mother and baby are really a biological unit. It is therefore essential to assess the mother also, and ask about her background, upbringing, and marriage. It can sometimes be useful to see the father as well.

Sir Robert Hutchinson once divided doctors into the 'wind-uppers' and the 'pooh-poohers', and some mothers too are like this, either exaggerating the symptoms or making light of them. This is particularly noticeable in the mothers of children with asthma. Here the doctor should be careful not to be misled but to turn for objective assessment to a peak-flow meter.

Perhaps the last question should be 'Have you any other worries you wish to discuss?', as there are often other unrelated problems about which the mother would welcome reassurance. These may be about something she does not wish the child to hear; if so, he can easily be sent out with the nurse for a short time.

Information from the child

Interviews proceed better if the child's eye level is at or even above the doctor's! (Only headteachers look down from behind a desk.) The child should be addressed using his own name and with a friendly smile and a soft confidential voice. Address him as an equal and in a manner appropriate to his age. A consultation is usually fairly serious, so avoid trying to be facetious.

A period of privacy with a child can be very revealing, especially if there is any question of psychosomatic or emotional disorder. A child will never tell you about non-accidental injury or incest in the presence of the parents. It is well worth while, therefore, to ask the child what *he* or *she* is worried about, as the child might have completely different worries from the mother. Histories taken from five-year-olds and those older can be better than the mother's! Give them a drawing book and a felt-tip pen and ask them to draw a dog or a house for this can tell you a lot about the child, and also often starts a conversation.

Suspected sexual abuse

A recent phenomenon which requires special attention is the remarkable increase in the referral of children with possible sexual abuse. As this is a new field there still remains much debate on how best to undertake the delicate and complex task of handling these cases in order (1) to find if a crime has occurred and (2) if the child needs protecting. The diagnosis of sexual abuse depends primarily on what the child has to say. So it is vital that the interviewing is done by an expert who understands the mind of a child and who has had training in this specialized field. Thus, multiple interviews by inexperienced people can be disastrous.

The interview must take place in a safe, relaxed setting and the interviewer (of either gender) must take time to build up a good rapport and be prepared to *listen* without pressuring the child into saying what the interviewer wants him/her to say. The duration and number of interviews must depend on many factors and especially the age of the child. It appears that children seldom lie about this subject though not every detail can be taken literally. So any statement about sexual abuse should be accepted until proven otherwise.

For further information on this extensive field the reader is referred to relevant publications [91,92].

Consultation with older children

In recent years, there have been legal problems over doctors being consulted by older children without the knowledge of their parents, or by those at variance with their parents over correct management. The Law Lords have now declared that doctors can institute treatment for children under the age of 16 years provided that the child has been properly informed and understands what is involved. Normally, parental approval should be sought, but there are occasional, unusual circumstances in which the doctor may be a better judge of what is best for the child's welfare than the parents. This increased recognition of the *child*'s rights should be approved of.

THE EXAMINATION

The co-operation of the child can make a great difference, so care must be taken from the outset to avoid upset. By the time this stage is reached, it is to be hoped that the family has got to know the doctor and that apprehension and anxiety have lessened.

The child should be respected as an individual in his own right and not moved around as if he were a plastic doll to be physically manipulated irrespective of his feelings. If clothing has to be removed, this is best done by the mother or, in an older child, by himself with instructions as to how much to take off. No one, not even a child, likes being undressed or being completely naked in front of a stranger. Underpants should be left on if possible. As soon as the examination is complete the child should be dressed again.

Any instruments to be used, such as a stethoscope or auriscope, should be demonstrated by using them on a teddy bear or by letting the child listen to his own heart sounds. It is useful to examine the heart, lungs, and abdomen first, as crying can seriously interfere with these examinations. Unpleasant procedures, such as ear and throat inspection, can be kept till last. Remember that tonsils can often be glimpsed without using a spatula.

A baby can best be examined on the mother's knee or on a couch, whereas toddlers are happier standing up beside their mother. There is no difficulty in feeling the abdomen in this way. Most children feel vulnerable and exposed when lying flat.

If any discomfort is likely, this should be explained first and assurance should be given that you will do your best not to hurt. Some children co-operate to a remarkable extent, but this depends on the child's nature and background. Even rectal examinations are usually well tolerated provided the finger is inserted very slowly to ease open the sphincter. The child should be told 'I'm just going to see what I can feel round here.'

Occasionally, however good the approach is, one meets with a child who totally resists physical examination and refuses to remove any article of clothing. The doctor should appreciate that this is not necessarily 'bloody mindedness', but that there are sometimes good reasons for this type of behaviour. Some such children may simply be fearful of what is to happen and one should respect this and try to allay their fears. Others may be manipulative or undisciplined, and here a firm no-nonsense approach may work. If unsuccessful, the doctor may have to decide whether any information that is likely to be gained justifies forcing the issue. This, in fact, is rarely necessary and to be considered only when there is a possibility of serious disease. In most cases, if the mother cannot persuade her child to co-operate, then it is best to leave matters and arrange a further visit. I remember a domiciliary visit when the child heard a doctor was coming and promptly locked himself into a garage at the bottom of the garden! I never saw him and the problem cleared up spontaneously after discussion with the parents.

REASSURANCE AND EXPLANATION

This is the most important part of the consultation: it is in fact what most parents have come for. The doctor will have considered the *whole* child and the environment, not just the disease, and will have made at least a provisional diagnosis, not a collection of alternatives. If the doctor is himself unsure about the diagnosis, then he should be frank with the parents and explain the situation to them.

Parents want to know why their child is ill. There is a common attitude that when things go wrong it is somebody's fault, so parents often need reassurance that they are not to blame. They also want to know what is best for their child, so a plan of action has to be formulated. Good communication with the mother, in the type of language that she understands, is essential, although the doctor should maintain a professional approach and not descend to vulgarity or familiarity.

It is futile to attempt reassurance by saying 'There is really nothing wrong', for the mother would not be there with her child if there were not a problem she wanted to be resolved.

Many common diseases, Henoch–Schönlein purpura for example, have never been heard of by most mothers, so a simple explanation of what is wrong must be given. If the symptoms and signs suggest a psychosomatic disorder, as in a child with recurrent abdominal pains, then time has to be spent discovering the environmental stress responsible and what can be done to relieve it. Remember to give some explanation to the child, too, as he has a right to know what is going on 'inside his tummy'. The psychotherapeutic effect of these explanations can be impressive.

From time to time, it is the doctor's sad duty to have to inform parents that there is something seriously wrong with their child, such as mental handicap or a fatal disease. Although this is a particularly distressing experience for the parents, the truth must be told simply and clearly, so that they are not in any doubt as to the situation. The issue has to be faced. Accurate wording is essential, such as the use of 'mental retardation' rather than 'a little slow'. Being too gentle and kind will mislead, since there is often resistance to acknowledging and accepting the full extent of the tragedy. Therefore, as soon as the diagnosis is certain—as, for example, of Down's syndrome—the senior clinician should see both parents together in conditions of privacy, and explain in simple terms the diagnosis and its significance, avoiding extensive detail at this stage. He should quietly express his concern and sympathy. After answering immediate questions, he can conclude by letting the parents know there will be further meetings later. It is not necessary to go into a lot of medical detail (say, of the type of leukaemia), but it is wise to offer a gleam of hope where possible, since this can help the parents to come to terms with the situation.

There can be a great variation in response to news of tragedy, especially to mental handicap. One mother said 'Poor bairn, we'll just have to make the best of it'. This, however, is the exception, as the prospect of a seriously ill or disabled child is naturally a heartbreak to the parents.

The child who has a serious illness

The pattern of childhood illness has changed over recent years. Quite a number of children suffer from prolonged and serious illness which may ultimately be fatal, e.g. neoplastic disease, cystic fibrosis, and serious heart disease among others. They may require prolonged and strenuous treatment. The question arises of how to handle the child and his family and what to say to them. A child under six years seems to have little real appreciation of the true nature of death and may have little fear of death. However, by 10 years, he or she may ask direct questions about the future and the possibility of dying. The child will see through any attempt to mislead so they must be answered seriously but as reassuringly as possible. Some children seem inclined to avoid asking questions but reach a tacit understanding with their parents that death is 'in the future'. However, it helps them when they speak about their illness to someone who can offer a positive, hopeful outlook. What children seem to want mainly is a quiet, loving companionship and a climate of security and normality. This is probably more important than what is actually said.

The parents themselves need to talk to someone about their feelings, either with other parents in the same predicament or with a doctor who works in this field. They often need time to take in the import of the diagnosis. The brothers and sisters may also ask questions and these too must be answered truthfully but offering hope. Siblings can feel jealous or neglected, worrying, perhaps, about their own health. They may also develop stress-related illnesses like asthma or eczema. Wooley *et al.* [93] provided an excellent detailed account of how best to impart bad news to the family, and to offer them the information and support they require.

ARRANGEMENTS AT THE END OF THE INTERVIEW

Before the mother and child depart, the need for another interview may arise. A visit to a hospital, perhaps some distance away, can be a wearisome business for a young mother with many family commitments. Further surveillance, if necessary, can often be carried out by the family doctor. Some mothers may express a desire for a return visit though the doctor may not feel it is necessary; if the mother feels the need for this, it should be arranged.

Occasionally, it is apparent at the return visit that the parents have not complied with the doctor's recommendations. He should not be upset or angry, but should find out why this has happened, as there may be a reasonable explanation. The home may be chaotic, the mother depressed, or the child quite undisciplined and unco-operative. Non-compliance is certainly not unusual and doctors should appreciate this.

Many popular books on child care have appeared in America and Britain in the past eighteen years, indicating that parents feel the need for guidance that is not being provided by the health professions. In addition, there is now a great number of voluntary societies dealing with specific handicaps, e.g. Down's syndrome, Turner's syndrome, cystic fibrosis, mental handicap, spasticity, muscular dystrophy, brittle bones, spina bifida, and so on. These societies all publish booklets and arrange meetings so that mothers can be better informed and supported in the heavy task of caring for their children. All this complements what the doctor has attempted to explain to them. Fully informed parents can help their children much more than those left in uncertainty or ignorance.

Talking to adolescents

R.M. WRATE

Adolescents, because of their particular developmental concerns and vulnerabilities, present doctors with special problems in communication. Because of the proximity of their own adolescence, medical students can tune in to what an adolescent is saying much more readily than an older doctor. But this close identification with adolescents' attitudes and concerns can make it much more difficult for the student to form an objective, detached assessment of the extent and nature of problems within families. By and large, they are a healthy group; medical contact is more likely to arise as a result of psycho-social problems than from physical illness. Apart from the regular medical consultations associated with the treatment of chronic disorders, such as juvenile diabetes, rheumatoid arthritis, sensory impairment, and so on, the physical conditions in adolescents for which medical advice is most frequently sought are glandular fever, traumatic injury, and pregnancy. However, the last two are often associated with psycho-social problems, and these also complicate, or contribute significantly to, the functional impairment of adolescents with chronic disability. For these reasons, it is important for all doctors to be aware of the common adverse psycho-social factors affecting adolescents, and also to have some understanding of adolescence as a developmental process.

THE ADOLESCENT PROCESS

Adolescence is sometimes seen as a particularly carefree time. For instance, Wordsworth wrote of the French Revolution, 'Bliss was it in that dawn to be alive. But to be young was very heaven!' For centuries, western European literature has provided rich illustrations of the memory or experience of adolescence, but also of the intense and ambivalent attitude towards it. For example: 'My thoughtless youth was winged with vain desires' (Dryden). Was Hamlet such an example? Caught between love and hate, between intense peer-group interest and the affections and rejections of his step-parent family, in some respects he struggled with adolescent problems more contemporary than those described in *Catcher in the Rye*. Many adolescents now grow up in single-parent or step-parent families, facing an uncertain future both in terms of family ties and prospective employment. Sometimes the 'Sweet wine of youth' (Rupert Brooke) is never so sweet as when it is mourned. But family malaise or repeated episodes of illness, perhaps associated with social dislocation or long-term unemployment, may be the dominant experience during adolescence; for some it may be the many years of selfless support they gave to a disabled parent or sibling.

So for many, adolescence may not be a romantic time, and the vicissitudes of life can obviously affect adolescents and their parents in equal measure. However, youth is envied for its assumption of immortality; in Hazlitt's words, 'No young man believes he shall ever die.' Such omnipotence contributes to the 'very heaven' of adolescence, and out of it springs the capacity for impetuous mistakes: 'Youth is a blunder; manhood is a struggle' (Disraeli); 'She bid me take love easy, as the leaves grow on the tree; but I, being young and foolish, with her would not agree' (Yeats); 'Youth's a stuff will not endure' (*Twelfth Night*). Adolescents are frequently impatient but in general they are also uncomplaining, and sociological studies show that few fundamentally challenge their family or adult values. Instead, the support some adolescent children provide for their demoralized mothers (e.g. with abusive or alcoholic husbands) sometimes seems unlimited, and is given at considerable personal cost. A disturbing feature of some care-giving by children or adolescents is that it is given without complaining. In general, adolescents do not seek out support for themselves except in acute crises—hence the under-reporting of deprivation, abuse, and sexual assault, and the development of 'hot-lines' and drop-in advisory centres. Arranging a medical consultation for oneself with a family general practitioner may be an important (and rather unusual) act of independence for an adolescent; it can also be a small sign of an adolescent in considerable difficulty.

Putting aside the external world of adolescents, psychoanalysts such as Anna Freud and Peter Blos argue that within adolescents' internal world there is emotional turmoil; even in the most normal families, adolescents are said to oscillate between emotional regression and emancipatory striving [94]. It is difficult to tell how far this applies to the majority. Although it certainly seems true of many disturbed adolescents [95], sociological studies of normal adolescents (in Britain by Coleman [96], in the United States by Offer and Offer [97] suggest that for most their teenage years are relatively smooth and that maturation is accomplished with little difficulty or undue stress. Psychoanalysts and sociologists alike agree that during adolescence most vestiges of childhood are lost and an adult role-identity is gradually established.

Identity formation, once the *sine qua non* of adolescent theory, is now regarded as a complex phenomenon that evolves over many years. For example, gender identity is established in early childhood [98]; a youngster's sexual role-identity begins with hormonal puberty, and development continues over many years. Erikson [99], a prominent American psychoanalyst, argued that the roots of an adult work-role identity are laid down in early school life, depending upon whether a child's initiative and achievements were adequately supported. But later studies (e.g. Rutter *et al.* [100] also emphasize the influence of secondary-school experience, the extent to which the family fosters an educational commitment, and the importance of the employment opportunities available locally.

Other aspects of emotional development are the growth of a capacity for intimacy and the ability to cope with being alone and acting independently. Without this, a person is neither able to trust others deeply, nor to relinquish their support. Although the foundations for both capacities are established in early childhood, the increased drives of adolescence (sexual, assertive, and emancipatory) and adolescents' wider social contacts offer renewed opportunities for the development of trust and emotional independence.

Adolescence, then, is not a single stage of development. For example, as all teachers and youth leaders recognize, 13-year-olds and 18-year-olds are at completely different psychological stages, though both are experiencing biological adolescence (i.e. from hormonal puberty to the full development of secondary sexual characteristics). Most children's relationships with their parents and other adults demonstrate an ambivalence that begins to emerge, sometimes quite suddenly, in early adolescence (about 13–15 years of age), evidenced by questioning, suspicion, rejection, or contempt of adult values and authority. However, by late adolescence (18 plus) much of the ambivalence has gone, and the pattern of values that will characterize their early adult lives is established. Early and mid-adolescent friendship patterns are often intense, replacing a youngster's close family attachments and providing companionship for exploring the world outside the family and school. With the greater emotional independence of late adolescence, less uncritical friendships based on a greater mutuality of interests are possible.

It is also important to remember that there is enormous individual variation in adolescent development. In part, this is attributable to the variable timing of hormonal puberty, and in part it is gender-determined (girls' biological and psycho-social development is about two years in advance of boys', and they are much more preoccupied than boys with emotional issues). Adolescents are extremely sensitive to this variation, and so early and late developers often describe quite different adolescent experience (e.g. Weatherley [101]).

Considerable variation also arises as a result of family and cultural factors. For example, neurotic family functioning, chronic disability, or economic dependence may all promote and prolong emotional dependence upon the family long after biological adolescence has passed. Adolescent questioning or rejection of adult values and authority is uncommon in Muslim communities, and in cultures where occupational and economic advancement is dependent upon family influence. For cultural reasons, gender-role expectations in particular may vary and, to communicate effectively with adolescent patients and their families, doctors must respect and show sensitivity to these various cultural patterns. This is particularly difficult, but especially necessary, where an adolescent patient seems caught between two different identifications, that of their ethnic minority and that of the majority culture; taking sides may be difficult to resist, but is not often helpful.

Finally, to communicate effectively with adolescents and their families, it is useful to have some knowledge of the contemporary interests and concerns of adolescents, and the common expectations of them held by school, parents, further education colleges, youth training schemes, and so on. One is also at an unnecessary disadvantage if common assumption about youth problems are accepted uncritically. For example, in mid-adolescence, sexually active youngsters are far outnumbered by those who are sexually uncertain, and habitual alcohol abuse is far more frequent than the non-prescription use of drugs. It is also important to have some awareness of contemporary trends as they affect adolescence, e.g. adolescents' frequent involvement in part-time work in their last year or two at school, which increases their economic independence, widens their social world, and offers opportunities for the rehearsal of adult work-roles.

BASIC INTERVIEWING GUIDELINES

The first principle is always to recall that, despite their legendary existential dilemmas, adolescents are rarely solitary. Except for isolated and unemployed youngsters drifting through bed-and-breakfast or bed-sit accommodation, no adolescent lives alone in the full sense of the word. Those not living within a family may have long-standing involvement with a social work department or be supported by and well known to hostel staff. Schools, recreational interests, part-time jobs, or further education all offer opportunities to build up peer relationships in addition to those provided by friends and siblings. However, medical consultations are typically conducted on a one-to-one basis, taking adolescents out of their familiar group settings. Much of this chapter, therefore, deals with communicating with adolescents on an individual basis, but those who habitually work in this field are also aware of the advantages of talking to adolescents in a group setting.

Within social welfare provision, these group settings might be some form of residential living experience, or group meetings held in a local authority office or neighbourhood premises. Within adolescent psychiatric services, the most common setting is a family interview, which all those living at home, in addition to the patient, are invited to attend [95]. This permits an independent view of the adolescent's family, and allows family members to give their individual perspectives on the adolescent and on family relationships. For many adolescents, it is also less anxiety-provoking than being seen on their own. In an individual consultation, the adolescent or the doctor often feels stuck for words, but the presence of the adolescent's family offers frequent opportunities to re-direct questions to others, and to invite family views on the concern that the adolescent may have obvious difficulty in talking about [102]. This setting also permits brothers and sisters to volunteer often very useful information; sibling altruism rather than rivalry is the norm at most family interviews, however competitive or difficult sibling relationships were alleged to have been.

Adolescents often want to talk about their health concerns on their own, and may be reluctant to accept the presence of certain family members, even where behavioural or relationship difficulties are being discussed. However, there is little point in continuing with an individual consultation if it feels very awkward and seems to bear little fruit. In these circumstances, it is better to voice the need to talk to others or meet with them, and state it as a need rather than a request.

Some adolescents find it much easier to talk of their emotional problems in growing up or having to make the best of adverse upbringings by sharing these experiences with other adolescents in a group. A one-to-one consultation with a doctor can be quite intimidating, and it does not offer the opportunity for healthy adolescent identifications or so readily facilitate mutual problem-solving. Adolescents with chronic disabilities, e.g. juvenile diabetes, can benefit enormously from talking about their predicaments and adolescent experience in a group of similarly affected youngsters, where the doctor or other health professional acts as a group facilitator rather than as a problem-solver.

The second principle of successful communication with adolescents is that communication should take place within a relationship, rather than from a detached stance. Adolescents do not have the same experience of relating to strange adults as their parents do; nor are they accustomed to adopting the multiple social roles that adults have to take. In consequence, they may bring a freshness to their contact with a doctor, but are also likely to fall back on stereotyped perceptions and responses. They are likely to be particularly influenced by their previous contact with doctors and other authority figures, and by their experience of previous confiding relationships. For example, their perception of authority figures may be that they are assumed to act in arbitrary, unexplained, or insensitive ways. The success of previous confiding relationships (with parents, neighbouring adults or relatives, guidance teachers, and so on) will also affect adolescents' attitude towards a consultation. It is sometimes quite useful to ask about such experiences in the early part of an interview, as it will not only help the doctor become aware of these factors but will also convey to the adolescent patient the doctor's sensitivity to these experiences.

Some form of relationship-building at the beginning of the interview is consequently most important. Even a few questions about family, school, personal interests and career intentions, previous contact with hospitals and doctors, and so on, helps adolescents to feel they are being approached as a person. Adolescents are particularly sensitive to being patronized by adults, so this enquiry must be genuine rather than a ritual. Thus, the adolescent's perception of the doctor is an important aspect of the doctor–patient relationship; it is helpful if the doctor is felt to be a person too. An 'opaque' doctor (betraying little or nothing of himself as a person) will be perceived as insensitive and unlikely to listen, and may seem quite frightening. On the other hand, deliberate self-revelation is often seen by adolescents as patronizing or exhibitionistic. Thus, an attitude that conveys interest, concern, and egalitarianism without relinquishing personal authority is the important ingredient of relationship-building with adolescents, rather than any simple prescribed behaviour.

The third principle is that communication is more than simply talking. The talking should convey a sense of being related to as a person, and a sense of the adolescent's predicament being understood. This may be conveyed by the doctor taking some essential action as a consequence of what he has learnt, or by his helping the adolescent to make a difficult decision (e.g. about a pregnancy termination), or even by simply listening to the adolescent's predicament without being propelled into the sort of abrupt action or problem resolution that the adolescent's parents might feel driven to. Communication is thus about something being shared, about mutual involvement, and in the context of a medical consultation of something important being shared, whether it be a painful feeling, a frightening thought or health anxiety, or a difficult decision.

Communication is a multi-level information exchange; it is not simply confined to words. As Flaubert put it in *Madame Bovary*, 'Language is like a cracked kettle on which we beat out times for bears to dance to, while all the time we long to move the stars to pity.' Words are given added meaning by the grammatical syntax that governs their use, by the tone of voice in which they are spoken, and by non-verbal aspects of communication, e.g. facial expression, hand or body gesture, and eye contact or its absence. Words may be used in response to some communication, or to block communication, e.g. by a torrent of words or by a direct avoidance or disqualification of what someone else has said. Communication may be largely non-verbal, e.g. an adolescent may feel included in the communication between a doctor and his parents if intermittent eye contact with the adolescent is preserved.

Adolescents and their families may find it difficult to put certain feelings into words; the doctor might convey understanding by an empathic silence rather than by words, although it is always helpful for patients when a doctor is able to put difficult feelings into words. This might be as tentative as 'I guess there is something very difficult/upsetting you're/everybody's feeling just now', or 'Would you like me to help you make a decision about this?' In each instance, the doctor is trying to put into words the unspoken concerns emerging from the interaction between himself and the adolescent patient and/or his family.

The fourth principle is that there usually is a symmetry to interpersonal communication. Direct observation of interviews (e.g. by videotape recording) reveals not only how people mirror each other's non-verbal behaviour during a conversation, but also how the form of speech or questions also shapes responses [103]. For example, information-seeking questions tend to elicit information rather than affect, whilst affective responses are most frequently elicited by questions framed specifically to evoke them, e.g. 'How do you feel about all these illnesses your family has had in the last year? And what was it like for you?' With unforthcoming adolescents, an interviewer is often tempted to adopt a multiple-choice type question approach. Although this can be quite successful in getting some communication going, the answers often mirror the questions in both form and content, and quite a lot of subsidiary questioning may be necessary to establish the validity of the adolescent's responses. Conversely, a doctor may discover at the end of an interview with a patient that they did not talk at all about an issue they had previously intended to cover. It quite often turns out that the doctor has unwittingly mirrored the patient's avoidance of the issue. Again, at a non-verbal level, it is more difficult to establish rapport and empathy with adolescents who themselves relate poorly; warm or engaging youngsters elicit warmth and interest in themselves from others, whilst a sullen or hostile adolescent characteristically evokes negative responses from adults, and it often takes quite an effort not to react in this way.

COMMON PROBLEMS IN COMMUNICATION WITH ADOLESCENTS

First, from the adolescents' point of view, probably their most frequently voiced complaint is of not being listened to; adults may seem in a hurry or appear just to be looking for certain answers, or only listening for what they want to hear. The second most frequently voiced complaint probably is how often a conversation turns into unsolicited advice or a mini-lecture. Either of these situations would lead adolescents to feel they were not being taken seriously, and that the doctor was not interested in their individual viewpoints or any initiatives they may be contemplating (which may be true). There are five less common, though recurring, criticisms or complaints. The first is that of being patronized. Second, the doctor seems to side with the parents, either not taking the part of the adolescent, or colluding with the parents against him or her. Third, adults are 'nosey' (i.e. intrusive). Fourth, the adolescent does not understand the questions being asked: the words used are 'too big' or the sentences are too complex, or double negatives are used. Finally, the adults lack humour. This last point is important because humour is quite important to adolescents, allowing them to talk jokily between themselves about difficult subjects that otherwise would be too embarrassing, painful, or frightening to talk about in more direct way.

It is to be hoped that, with experience, a sensitive adult would not keep repeating many of these mistakes. Even for a sensitive doctor, the criticism most difficult to avoid might be the complaint of intrusiveness, since a doctor's role requires an enquiring approach. This difficulty, and the complaint of pro-parental bias, can be minimized by making it clear at the outset of the consultation that the adolescent is being seen in his or her own right (rather than, for instance, as the troublesome offspring of their parents) and by emphasizing that the doctor is interested in hearing about things from his or her point of view. Adolescents' complaints about 'nosiness' usually reflect strivings for independence rather than paranoid sensitivity. They usually do want to put adults into the picture, but do not welcome the regression (that is, to say dependency) that they assume from their childhood experience has to go with it.

DOCTORS' PERCEPTIONS

The two complaints most frequently voiced by doctors about adolescent patients are that they are unforthcoming or that they are sullen and hostile. In either case they are considered difficult to relate to, so that little effective communication takes place. Even where the parents have predicted this sort of difficulty, it is wise for the doctor to check that his own attitude (in the terms of the preceding section) has not unwittingly contributed to the impasse. Where it has, it is useful to acknowledge the fact, for example by saying 'I'm sorry, I was in a bit of a rush at the beginning. Can you tell me a bit more about what is upsetting *you?*' When the doctor shows that an error can be recognized and admitted, the adolescent's stereotyped picture of doctors is countered, and this alone may free things up. Since most silence and most sullenness is defensive, the particular value of an apology is that it reveals the doctor's concern for the patient and his dilemma, and for discovering the truth, rather than being interested in superiority or control. For the sullen or silent patient, it is especially important to build up a relationship before probing too much. If communication does get stuck, it is usually advisable to switch for a while to a more neutral line of enquiry, which can help to develop the relationship further.

When sullenness or hostility persists despite these efforts, it is usually safe to assume that it is a character trait rather than a specific response to the particular situation (e.g. because the patient has been forced to see the doctor against his wishes). Under these circumstances, the patient's manner should be alluded to during the questioning. The timing of this confrontation (see p. 48) and the degree of directness is important; for example, 'I

can see you're quite angry. Does this sometimes get in the way of
. . . remembering to take your tablets/test your urine/follow advice
about diet', and so on. In each example, the anger is referred to as
a possible problem *for the adolescent*, but this controlled approach
can be difficult if the adolescent's negativism has got under the
doctor's skin. Once again, it is best to acknowledge openly when
this has occurred, especially if it has happened to such a degree
that the doctor no longer feels he can evince much interest in
the adolescent's views: for example, 'Look, I'm finding it very
difficult to help you when I'm getting so mad at you—can you
stop . . . drinking that Coke/kicking the table/talking to me like
that?' This approach may be of equal value with a bullying or
intimidating patient: 'I'm not going to be able to help you if you
get me frightened of disagreeing with you' or 'I'll not be able to
think straight, and that's no good to you. So can you cut out the
threats?'

The persistently silent adolescent calls for a different approach.
On the whole, such patients are much more difficult to deal with,
because it is often difficult to tell what is causing the silence. It
might be unhappiness, depression, demoralization, anxiety, or
perhaps severe embarrassment. It might equally be distrustfulness
or an unspoken hostility, and some adolescent patients give barely
an indication as to which of these it might be. The best places to
look for clues in deciphering the silence are in the history that
is available, and in the doctor's own emotional responses. For
example, social withdrawal and tearfulness in the presence of loss
of appetite and weight suggest depression, but in their absence
suggest some form of phobic anxiety state. Either condition calls
for a lot of patience, which is usually not difficult to find, and the
doctor can put into tentative words what he believes the patient
might be feeling but finding difficult to express; for example, 'I
guess you're feeling quite/rather unhappy/helpless/hopeless at the
moment. Can you tell me a bit about that?' If from the history
there are reasons to suppose the patient has difficulty (perhaps
justifiably) in trusting others, this needs to be included in some
way in what is said; for example, one might add to the comment
above 'You may find I understand you a bit more than you would
expect me to!'

If during the consultation with a silent, seemingly unhappy
adolescent, the doctor finds himself becoming *unusually* irritated

or angry, this can be important, if indirect, evidence of a strong unspoken negativism on the patient's part. Once the doctor has checked that his reaction is not some displaced anger of his own, e.g. with a colleague, another patient, or a relative, it is best to make reference to the anger as if it originated with the patient. For example, 'I wonder if it's hard to talk at the moment because of how angry you're feeling?' If the patient denies anger or asks why the question was asked one can reply 'I was just feeling that' or 'I just guessed.' The denial does not mean the doctor was wrong, and the patient may be relieved that the doctor asked the question, endorsing the disclosure of angry feelings. Further silences can be handled by taking a one-down position; for example, 'A few minutes ago I was wondering if you were feeling . . . Can you help me understand what's upsetting you?'

It does not help the adolescent patient to allow his persistent silence to control the consultation. If no real progress is occurring, it is better to draw the consultation to a close than to prolong it further. The doctor is then left with two choices: either to see the patient again (without undue delay) or to arrange a further appointment that includes one other family member. At this point, it is usually a mistake to give the patient the choice, as this option is generally used as another opportunity to express negativism. Instead, the doctor should follow his own gut feeling, remembering that some of these silent patients will feel disappointed if they are not given a second chance to talk on their own.

CONFIDENTIALITY

Finally, a note on *confidentiality* as it applies to adolescents. Most patients, whatever their age, talk more freely if they feel that what they say will go no further than the doctor to whom they are speaking. On the other hand, most of these patients simultaneously wish that their relatives better understood their predicament, and in the case of children and young adolescents such understanding is essential. A useful rule of thumb is to give adolescents an assurance of confidentiality that is modified in a single important respect: if by the end of the consultation something has been talked about that the doctor feels is essential for the adolescent's parents to know, then the parents must be told. The patient and doctor can then discuss what and how the parents are told, but not whether they are told. Almost without exception, adolescents find this acceptable, and rarely seem inhibited by the conditional nature of the confidentiality.

OTHER SPECIFIC PROBLEMS

A number of additional problems need to be reviewed briefly: the suicidal adolescent; adolescents complaining of sexual abuse; patients with anorexia nervosa; adolescents with chronic medical disorders; oppositional or rebellious adolescents; and adolescents estranged from their families or experiencing severe family disruption.

Parasuicide

As a form of communication, parasuicidal behaviour should always be taken seriously [104]. One must assume that the underlying distress is genuine, however outwardly histrionic it seems, and that the adolescent feels in an otherwise insoluble predicament. The parasuicidal behaviour is a maladaptive solution, albeit an impulsive one and perhaps modelled on another's behaviour. Aside from the assessment of further suicidal risk in the immediate future, there are two principal tasks in talking with these adolescents. First, to try to understand their predicament, as far as is possible, from their point of view; second, to remind them gently of the unfortunate consequences of parasuicide—how would their families feel if they had succeeded?—and to help them identify some initial steps towards resolution of their problems. A response of 'I don't care' from the adolescent should not deter the doctor from reminding such patients that they have responsibilities whether they like to think of them or not.

Sexual abuse

Intra-familial sexual abuse is now known to be much more common than was once thought [105]. Three factors inhibit adolescents from talking about it: shame, guilt, and the (sometimes quite justified) fear that disclosure would break up the family. For these reasons, some sexually abused adolescents may be terrified if asked directly whether it has occurred, but the vast majority will also feel immensely relieved that the abuse has finally come out into the open. For those for whom the sexual abuse is still occurring, the revelation of the guilty secret may offer the first tangible hope of its stopping. In talking with such adolescents, four issues need to be addressed. First, the patient's shame and guilt. Second, how those involved in the adolescent's care should be informed, and any practical steps that need to be taken to ensure the adolescent is not at risk of further abuse. Third, preserving the adolescent's future relationship with the doctor. Fourth, the family's probable reactions to the allegation, which invariably include strenuous denial whatever the truth. Quite often the adolescent faces being excluded from the family. Because of these problems, the veracity of the adolescent's account should not be doubted simply on the basis of some inconsistency or later retraction [106].

To help adolescents come to terms with their feelings of shame and guilt, it is essential to point out the universality of their emotional response, and to remind them emphatically that as child victims of adult misbehaviour they were not responsible for what took place. Guilt is to be expected, but it is inappropriate. Often it is also necessary to spend some time letting them express their anger with the perpetrator and their resentment that their mother or family had not discovered and put a stop to the abuse, particularly since, in most instances, the adolescent will have tried several times before to draw attention to the situation. The adolescent may also wish to talk in detail about what took place. It is often not easy to tolerate listening to these outpourings of feelings and memories, and the impulse to cut off the adolescent's account or reveal one's own feelings, or take some other precipitate action is often strong. In each case these impulses should be resisted and time given instead for reflection, which includes considering how the disclosure might affect the patient's future relationship with the doctor. For instance, the perpetrator may also be a patient of the same doctor. Perhaps of greater importance, it may be difficult for adolescents to return to the doctor after disclosing so much about themselves. If the doctor feels this could be the case, he can help matters by clearly indicating that this is something he would wish to avoid: for example, 'I know it wasn't easy telling me what happened, and I suppose you'll now have quite mixed feelings about having done so—I hope that doesn't make it hard for you to come back and see me next week.'

Anorexia nervosa

Adolescents with anorexia nervosa call for a special approach, as it is easy to fall in with their massive, though denied, dependency needs. They resent it intensively if the doctor treats them as children by (for example) offering vague reassurance that cannot be backed up, or medication with no clear purpose, by by-passing the adolescent when talking with her invariably distraught parents, or by not giving her a chance to talk to the doctor on her own. Whatever the individual factors responsible for the condition, a striking feature is how often anorexia nervosa constitutes a developmental moratorium, or even a wholesale retreat from growing up. Emancipatory strivings for control then become increasingly channelled into anorexic preoccupations; underneath the anorexic adolescent's controlling behaviour, her self-esteem is usually very low and her identity fragile [107]. Emotional over-involvement and habitual conflict–avoidance are common features of the families of anorexic patients. In responding to the difficulties of the patient and her family, it is important for their doctor not simply to mirror, i.e. repeat, the patient's or the family's behaviour by reacting with similar anxiety-driven counter-control, which would readily stifle any quite appropriate but tentative bids for independence on the part of the patient.

Adolescents with chronic medical disorders

A major problem during the adolescence of many youngsters with chronic disorders is the struggle they have to establish a sense of self-reliant competence and emotional independence in the face of their ongoing physical limitations and their continued enforced dependence upon their parents and health-care professionals. The oscillating pattern of child-like regression and emancipatory striving referred to earlier is frequently seen in this patient group. Much emotional or behavioural disturbance in these youngsters centres around this single issue, even when adolescents are apparently well adjusted to their disability. During a consultation, the doctor's role may quite often be to reinterpret the patient's complaints in these terms, and to recognize opportunities to foster a true sense of competence in the patient. With these particular adolescents, the doctor's stance might be best described as a consultant to the 'executive', enabling the adolescents to become as much in charge of themselves as possible.

The oppositional adolescent

Underlying, or indeed driving, the posture of rebellion and indifference to adult authority and values shown by these youngsters, there is often the opposite—they are struggling with very strong dependency needs. They become most oppositional with adults who matter to them, although sometimes they may treat all adults in the same way, as they attribute to symbols and figures of authority the characteristics of arbitrary inflexibility. Viewing adult power in this light, these adolescents feel that they can maintain their own identity only if they challenge that power. In general, therefore, these adolescents require a gentle approach. Where possible their outspokenness should be accepted without rebuke; their aggressive stance and comments should be ignored or turned by humour; and their concerns should be listened to with respect. Often this is the converse of what they have come to expect (particularly from their families) and most of these adolescents respond favourably, their gratitude being unspoken but none the less evident. Any recrudescence of rudeness can then be much more easily dealt with; for example, by the doctor reminding them how much easier it is for him to help them when he is not being sworn at or shouted at.

Family disruption and estrangement

Although much has been written on this subject and how to deal with it by using family therapy techniques [102,108], comments here will be confined to what is particularly applicable to brief consultations, either with the adolescent alone or with the parent(s). In general, it takes two to have a quarrel, and parents often unwittingly contribute to the difficulties they complain of by being over-critical or restrictive, *laissez-faire* or disinterested, sulking, or in other ways undermining the adolescent's moves towards independence.

In order to understand what has been going wrong, it is therefore essential to get full and exact details of at least one of the crises being complained of, rather than allowing oneself to be flooded with complaints of a general kind. It is also important during the interview to convey to family members one's own impartiality and readiness to listen to the viewpoint of all concerned. Once the family members have been listened to, it is their turn to listen; if any advice given is then not followed through, they have less cause for complaint.

With some estranged adolescents and their families, the task is a different and often more difficult one: helping them gradually to accept one another's limitations. For a few, this may mean living independently, either as an immediate necessity or as a long-term requirement.

SUMMARY

Despite the many difficulties described in this chapter, talking with adolescents is usually rewarding, since most are lively, curious, and hopeful that their concerns will be taken seriously. Because they are in transition from childhood, their dependency needs are still great and their family identifications are strong. Thus, adults remain extremely important figures in the lives of most young people, even though at times they and their parents may doubt that this is so. There is, however, considerable variation in psychological development during adolescence, partly a result of biological factors and partly related to socio-cultural influences.

Previous experience of confiding relationships, both familial and extra-familial, are particularly important influences, and will certainly affect how adolescents respond to any medical consultation. Some may welcome the opportunity to speak alone, while others find this intimidating and feel at ease only if a relative or their family is present. In whichever way they are met, some initial relationship-building is an important step, and good continued communication is dependent upon a good relationship being preserved thereafter. This is especially true for those youngsters for whom it was the parents, or other adults, who were responsible for the consultation taking place.

A non-patronizing attitude and a preparedness to listen are vital.

Attention should be paid to non-verbal aspects of communication, and to the manner of what is said as well as to the words. At times this may include relying on one's intuitive understanding of the adolescent, and scrutinizing one's own emotional reactions. Where possible, it is generally helpful to maintain an attitude of hopefulness and an expectation of finding positives in the adolescent. For example, just as most adolescents welcome sharing their predicaments with a doctor whom they would regard as a trusted adult, so do most adolescents respond well when of necessity the doctor in turn decides to share with them a predicament in which the youngster has placed the doctor; say, by wanting the doctor not to tell their parents that they are 18-weeks pregnant. Talking to the adolescent then becomes mutual problem-solving, rather than something that is 'done to' the adolescent.

Talking to the elderly

C.T. CURRIE

The past is another country, from which there are visitors among us. They are the elderly. For them, many things are different: money,* transport, communications, newspapers, public and private behaviour, even the landscape of the streets. Most older people have adapted quite well to the gradual transition from the familiarities of the period in which their attitudes were formed, but young people dealing with elderly patients should at least be aware of just how much change is involved.

People in their twenties today who are looking after people almost as old as the century should know that in their generation childhood death from infectious illness was commonplace, that the men could have been among the younger participants in the First World War, and that the women were among the first to have the vote. In their young adulthood, jazz was new, cars were rare, doctors were expensive and largely ineffective visitors to their homes, divorce was extremely unusual, employment was hard to come by, and housework was for most a gruelling and messy business. Whether as civilians or as servicemen and women, they have endured the rigours of two world wars. And to keep the generation gap in perspective, it is also worth remembering that the 80-year-olds of the 1920s were survivors from the early Victorian era.

Generalizations about the elderly abound, but few of them withstand rigorous inspection. There is perhaps one exception, illustrated by the life of a distant relative of mine. Great-aunt Kate was born in the 1870s. A woman of some spirit, she was an active suffragette in the early part of this century. Later, when women drivers were still very unusual, she was a 'prominent lady

---

* Two elderly women were overheard discussing the decimalization of British currency in 1972: 'They should have waited until all the old people died off before they changed the money.'

motorist'. She raised a family and was widowed and re-entered local politics and caused consternation as one of a minority who welcomed a proposed Polaris base in the early 1960s. When she was 99 and still living alone in a bungalow she had occupied for 60 years, she became somewhat frail and accepted the services of a home help. When she was 101, she showed signs of senile dementia and became more dependent, eventually entering a nursing home. She died at the age of 102. If there is a generalization about old age, it might be that the second hundred years is tougher!

The diversity of the elderly is the principal attraction in being involved in their care. Any randomly selected group of old people will demonstrate a huge range of physical and mental preservation, of personality, and of life history. Most old people are easy to communicate with, a few less so. Barriers to communication are worth learning about, and the acquisition of a little understanding and a few basic skills is a simple and a rewarding exercise. Although most old people are well, the presence in the health-care system of a small percentage of a very large number—nine million British citizens are of pensionable age—means that in most specialties many or even most clinical encounters are with the elderly.

ATTITUDES TO THE ELDERLY

Unfortunately, the education of health-care professionals does not reflect this demographic reality. In teaching hospitals, the older patient may be seen as some kind of marginally acceptable substitute for the real thing. Surgical wards and acute medical units may persist with an internalized model of a bygone age when patients had the courtesy to be young and the wisdom to present with only one diagnosis. The challenge of an inexorable shift towards the provision of acute services for an elderly out-patient and in-patient clientele may still be met with puzzlement or denial of the reality of the problem.

For older health professionals, whose training took place and whose attitudes were formed before the rise of geriatric medicine and its incorporation into medical and other health professional training, all this can be particularly stressful. Uneducated in the nuances of presentation and challenges of the management of disease in the elderly, and bewildered by the complex interrelationships of the physical, psychological, and social difficulties of some elderly patients, they may patronizingly over-simplify matters by talking about 'social admissions' or succumb to the temptation of defending a specialty defined as narrowly as possible and speak and write indignantly of 'bed-blockers'.

Such habits of mind among seniors are easy for juniors to perceive and hard for them to resist. Interestingly, there is evidence that the most junior medical students have attitudes towards the elderly that are more favourable than those of their senior student and junior hospital doctor colleagues. It appears that teaching hospitals have at present a negative effect on students' attitudes to the elderly, although ther is also evidence that formal teaching about the special needs and potential of the elderly patient can reverse this. In other words, if you know how to sort out the problems of your older patients, you will feel happier about dealing with them. This dissemination of a positive attitude towards the care of the elderly is probably the major achievement of the expansion of undergraduate teaching of geriatric medicine in Britain over the last eighteen years.

COMMON BARRIERS TO COMMUNICATION WITH THE ELDERLY

Dementia

This condition, particularly in its lesser degrees, is common in elderly patients. Around 10 per cent of over-65s have irreversible mental impairment, severe in around a half of the cases. About 25 per cent of over-85s are affected. Surveys of patients in the care of general practitioners and hospital doctors have shown that dementia is poorly recognized. Although the condition is untreatable, it is well worth recognizing and assessing, because some reversible confusional states masquerade as dementia, and because dementia, if present, affects the further management of the case in many ways. It is wise when dealing with an elderly patient to assume the presence of mental impairment until tactful but effective testing has confirmed or excluded it.

Because most doctors are in a hurry most of the time, and because patients respond badly to some of the more elaborate and less socially acceptable forms of mental testing (such as being asked to count backwards from 20 or to repeat gnomic sentences about a nation's supply of wood), the following test is recommended. Ask the patient her age, and then her year of birth, and then, perhaps with some gentle introduction such as 'And now, just to test your memory', what year it is now. This test is brief, non-disruptive, and has the great advantage of being independent of external verification and involving only a little arithmetic well within the capacity of most doctors!

If a patient scores three out of three on this simple test, there is for all practical purposes no serious problem. One, two, or three mistakes, or straightforward incomprehension, have proportionate significance. There is no point in embarking on a detailed and complex clinical history from a demonstrably severely impaired patient. Other sources of information will have to be found. Dementia (or, less commonly, a reversible confusional state) has been demonstrated.

Undiagnosed mental impairment can cause great problems for the patient and all concerned with her. A vague but socially well-preserved old lady will react to close clinical questioning like a slippery witness, because she does not want to admit that she does not know. 'Which came first? The pain or the sickness?' 'What——?' 'But you said the sickness only a moment ago.' The truth is that she can remember neither the sequence of events nor what she has just said, and that time spent on further detailed questioning will be wasted. A few present-tense questions such as 'Are you in pain now?' and 'Does it hurt when I press you there?' will be useful in almost any circumstances, but time will be saved and frustration, embarrassment, and sometimes even risk, will be avoided by evaluating the mental state before almost any other enquiry.

The doctor assessing a mentally impaired elderly patient now has two additional tasks: to determine the nature and severity of the deficit, and to ascertain from other sources the information that would, in the absence of the deficit, have been obtainable. But to have recognized the problem of mental impairment and to have documented it will promote realism in further communication with and about the patient and in the subsequent handling of the case.

Deafness

Around 25 per cent of people over the age of 75 years have hearing difficulties, ranging from mild impairment, in which a loud conversational voice is helpful, to total isolation from intelligible sound. Many elderly people are embarrassed as well as isolated by the disability and may attempt to conceal it by a mixture of lip-reading and bluff. If a patient gives unexpected bizarre or even just excessively bland answers, it is worth thinking about whether they have actually heard the question.

Deafness slows up history-taking and can create or allow misunderstanding. It can also cause embarrassment, as when intimate details of a clinical enquiry have to be shouted aloud within the earshot of others. It is a simple and considerate matter to ask a patient if he can hear you easily. If not, there are several simple measures that may help.

The first is to speak in a clear and loud conversational voice with one's face in full view of the patient. If you shout, consonants tend to get lost and vowel sounds are distorted. In some forms of deafness, shouting can cause discomfort verging on pain. A loud conversational voice, with clear lip movements to assist lip-reading, will help most. If the patient has a hearing aid, it makes sense to find it and to check its setting or indeed its batteries, as necessary. Some wards and clinics have light and easily used amplifiers, with earphones or 'wand' earpieces, that greatly facilitate communication with the deaf. If all else fails and you have to talk very loud or shout, try to do so in a closed room, out of the main ward or clinic area, to minimize embarrassment to the patient and inconvenience to others. If deafness is absolute and the patient has satisfactory vision, writing short questions on a large notepad is time-consuming but worthwhile for essential information.

Dysarthria

This is disordered articulation of speech. Language function is intact; that is, the patient can comprehend the spoken word and formulate speech and sound but has a difficulty, usually at the level of the pharynx, mouth, or lips, that makes speech slurred and indistinct. The most common cause is stroke disease which affects lip and tongue movements. Missing dentures are a less common cause. Various neurological disorders affecting the brainstem or cerebellum may also cause dysarthia.

A dysarthric interviewee is helped by patience, sympathy, and lack of embarrassment on the part of the interviewer. Persistence will be rewarded as the patient's particular problems with articulation become more familiar and speech becomes gradually more comprehensible. Where appropriate, finding the lost false teeth is an obvious and helpful thing to do, and will be much appreciated.

Dysphasia

This condition is an abnormality of language function usually caused by stroke damage to the left hemisphere. Around two-thirds of patients with right-sided weakness due to stroke show some evidence of dysphasia. In most cases, both receptive and expressive language functions are affected to some degree, i.e. the patient has difficulty both with deciphering sound into meaning and with encoding meaning into words. Since major loss of language can occur with good cognitive preservation, dysphasia can be a very distressing experience for the patient, who is aware of his world yet out of communication with it. Perhaps most distressing is the plight of the patient with a predominantly expressive dysphasia who is assumed also to be incapable of understanding speech. To be talked about, perhaps unsympathetically, by medical and nursing staff unaware that everything they say is being fully understood, could be a hideous experience for an alert and cognitively intact patient, combining anguish, frustration, and resentment. It is kindest and safest to assume understanding until the facts have been determined.

The approach to the dysphasic patient is at first diagnostic: which language functions have been affected, and to what degree and what, if any, cognitive impairment is also present? An alert-looking patient, behaving appropriately to his or her circumstances, is likely to be quite well-preserved mentally even if he or she cannot utter a word. Many smile and nod as though to initiate wordless encounter. Polite greetings—'Hello, good morning', etc., are visibly appreciated. Receptive function can be assessed quickly and reliably in the patient who cannot speak by asking him or her to perform a simple action such as putting out the tongue or raising the left hand. It is surprising how often that kind of request, intended to test purely language function, is spoiled for its true purpose by the inclusion of some non-verbal cue. A sympathetically phrased question about language function, such as 'Is it that you know what you want to say but can't put it into words?' may prompt an emphatic but wordless agreement, often also demonstrating relief that someone (at last?) knows how the patient feels.

The unlikeable elderly patient

Not all elderly patients are approachable, personable, and easy to get on with, and any realistic account of the problem of communicating with the elderly should recognize this. The rational handling of an encounter with an unlikeable patient begins with the recognition of one's own reactions. Only by being open to one's own less admissible feelings is it possible to handle them and remain both in control of oneself and helpful to the patient. The less attractive patient, the unpleasant patient, and the patient who is frankly not far short of ghastly are all still patients first and foremost, in need of care, assessment, and management, and, whatever one's initial reaction, just as much part of one's job as their less repellent fellows!

There is no doubt that unattractive patients are at risk for certain misfortunes. When doctors are busy, they are more likely to be left to the last. If it is possible to delegate, they will end up as the immediate responsibility of the most junior member of the team. In the day-to-day life of the ward, they become isolated and perhaps the recipients of less preferential nursing care.

The first step, then, in dealing with the unlikeable patient is to be aware of one's own reaction. Thereafter, the trick is to detach oneself a little from one's reaction, to work out why it is the patient seems unpleasant, and to proceed on the basis that the resulting information is an integral part of the assessment and perhaps also of some clinical significance.

Health professionals are for the most part reared in the traditions of middle-class cleanliness. A dirty patient, visually unpleasant and perhaps also malodorous, is more difficult for us to deal with than a clean one. It is tempting to back off, or to adopt a more abrupt or even a judgemental attitude. (One of my contemporaries in a casualty job used to ask such patients when they last had a bath, and sometimes even enquire solemnly when they were last in jail!) To retreat is contrary to the conditioning and instinct to care, and sets up anxiety. To be harsh is to betray trust or, in some cases, simply to reinforce previous low expectations on the part of the patient. Negligence that occurs because the patient is dirty and therefore escapes thorough examination is, of course, unforgivable. We can do better.

The key to preserving calmness and efficiency in relation to the dirty patient is to develop an active and enquiring attitude towards the problem of dirt. Why is the patient dirty? Is the dirt acute or chronic? The significance of ingrained grime, black-bordered fingernails, and long curly toenails is very different from that of a single episode of faecal incontinence. In the former case, self-neglect is likely to be related to dementia. Because of mental impairment, the patient has lost the insight and self-care capacity that keeps most of us fairly clean. Brief mental testing is the next step. In the latter case, it may be that an old lady has taken her laxative, fallen, broken her hip, lain overnight in fear and pain, and in the morning endured the humiliation of the first episode of incontinence she has experienced for seven or eight decades. The clinical significance of her offensive state, the result of temporary helplessness, is very different.

The same approach can be applied equally usefully to other components of unlikeability. The first step is to recognize one's emotions; the next is to identify just what it is that is upsetting about the patient; the third is to understand that identified factor in terms of its clinical significance. Thus, irritants are neutralized by turning them into more information about the patient, for further assessment and action as necessary.

Other presentations of dementia can be equally irritating or repulsive. There are old people with severe mental impairment who are almost 'professionally old', coming across as vain and repetitious and saying things like 'I'm 93 and I'm wonderful for my age' several times over a few minutes. They may well be vain, with little to be vain about. They are a lot more repetitious than they think they are, because they cannot recall having made their main conversational contribution only a few minutes or seconds before. Again, simple mental testing will objectify the problem and a moment's reflection will greatly increase one's sympathy for the patient's regular carers.

Another frequently unlikeable patient is the undiagnosed depressive, particularly one who is hypochrondriacal and poly-symptomatic. A screening instrument to aid the detection of depression in elderly medical in-patients has been described [130]. Many of these patients have previous adverse experience of medicine, low expectations, and high anxiety, all of which further diminish the prospects of an easy encounter. The moaning old woman with a sore back may have been seen in orthopaedic out-patients, have been found to have arthritis to a degree unremarkable for her age, and been given a corset that did not help much. Other minor chronic symptoms may have taken her to other single-system clinics, and she may be on a great many medications. She pours out a litany of luridly described phenomena which bear little relation to what we read of in textbooks. She answers simple questions with psychotic intensity: 'Do you have a headache?' 'Yes! Like a giant banging nails into my head.' 'Do you get indigestion?' 'Yes . . . Like wee red-hot golf balls jooglin' aboot in my stomach.'

A good way of remaining calm through such an interview is to write down as much as possible verbatim. The cumulative miseries crowded on the page are virtually diagnostic. It is easy to see why such patients are unpopular and why they are passed from clinic to clinic, but a few of the key questions concerning a possible depressive illness will take the case a lot further. Yes, the patient sleeps badly and wakes early. Yes, her mood is low and sometimes she wishes she were dead. She has depression and needs a trial of medication rather than exhaustive investigation of each and every symptom. An unlikeable patient has been transformed to one with a single, highly treatable illness!

The patient has benefited and so has the doctor. Such an active and diagnostic approach to the unlikeable patient is in everyone's interest. The guilt of delay or delegation can be avoided. A potentially frustrating, muddled encounter, which could have left the doctor feeling angry and impotent, can be transformed into an intellectually and professionally satisfying part of his or her work. Most of us would rather help patients than feel angry with them or helpless about their problems. Broadening one's clinical assessment to include the unpalatable is not simple good practical medicine, it is enlightened self-interest.

THE OLD PEOPLE OF TOMORROW

We are the old people of tomorrow, if we are lucky. Survival into old age is an achievement. The historically recent mass survival to old age now happening in industrialized countries is a triumph of growing affluence, of public health rather than of individual medical care. It raises new issues for health and social serives and has opened up a large debate about public policy and the funding of care. At a personal level, it means that young and middle-aged people involved in health care meet many elderly patients, their care being a large part of everyday work.

Our attitudes to the elderly people we meet are shaped by many factors, perhaps not least by our feelings about growing old ourselves. The high premium on visual attributes associated with youth—see any magazine or newspaper, almost any film or TV programme—does little to diminish these fears. A stereotype of ageing as the loss of one's attractiveness to others is the unconscious negative correlative behind every 'Page three girl', every Keanu Reeves poster. Are fears of such losses simply an aspect of a late-adolescent preoccupation with self-image? In middle age now myself, I cannot clearly remember. It seems, however, that unexamined personal vanity figures in it somewhere. We should not let so unworthy a preoccupation, however central to our being, take over to the extent of damaging a potentially helpful clinical relationship.

A more powerful series of anxieties concerns infirmity. It is worth stating and restating that many old people are well and active, happy and fulfilled, and that—for obvious reasons—those we see in hospitals are a sample with a very powerful bias towards the unwell. Old age is not synonymous with dementia, or immobility, or incontinence, or dependency on others. True, such things are more common in old age, especially extreme old age, but for every older person in any form of institutional care there are twenty at large doing much the same sort of thing as their younger fellow citizens.

The frail elderly, the confused, and the dependent threaten us as the dying threaten us: we fear to become them. The difficulty for the young person confronted by such patients while still developing professional knowledge, skills, and attitudes is that of maintaining empathy without succumbing to fearful, irrational over-identification—a process so threatening and exhausting that a further alternative, that of rejection, all too easily presents itself. A sense of perspective helps. Few of the old—unblushingly I repeat this—are pitiable and helpless. More reassuring still, age does not spring upon us swiftly and randomly (as do some of the other things medical students and others read about in textbooks and worry about in the stillness of the night). Old age is a privilege granted only to those who live a long time.

A 20-year-old talking to someone aged 80 and feeling threatened by the encounter might usefully play a few tricks with time, little mental exercises that take only a few moments but provide yet another set of perspectives that might help. The first is to ask: what was this person like when he or she was my age? When was that? What was going on in the world then? What has happened over the intervening years, the years in which they traversed, in a sense, the time gap now between us?

That helps because quite simply it makes us think of the person before us as not *always* having been old. 'People talk to me as if I've always been 86!' is a much-quoted complaint of the elderly patient, and an entirely valid one. If we can reconstruct, however sketchily, a human life stretching over the best part of a century for the patient sitting in front of us we will do better, far better, in the matter of trying to help whatever is bothering them now. A few minutes spent with the patient on that theme, perhaps talking about work, family, and social conditions, will reward both participants: understanding and sympathy will be established before the narrow agenda of the formal clinical interrogation begins.

And there is another 60-year gap that is worth thinking about: the next 60 years in the life of the younger person in the encounter. Old age is not arrived at by crossing a line, though milestones like decade birthdays and retirement are undoubtedly noted. Old age will be reached via a series of broadly identifiable stages—young adulthood, maturity, middle age, late middle age—each marked by its own achievements, commitments, rewards, disappointments, and so on. Time will pass. Goals will change. Old age, if we are lucky, will one day be ours too. We cannot catch it from patients. We acquire it for ourselves, and it is nothing to be afraid of. Indeed there is much to be said for it. In the words of Maurice Chevalier, 'Old age isn't so bad—when you consider the alternatives'.

17 Talking to the dying patient

D. DOYLE

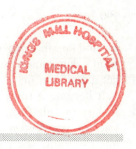

Those who are dying, contrary to what one might expect, seldom want their diagnosis discussed or repeatedly explained. But they *do* ask, in one way or another, for confirmation that they are dying; they are then ready to tackle the business in hand, that of living out what is left of life with minimal suffering, with a dignity that is defined by them and respected by their attendants, and with an unclouded mind. As death approaches, whether they are young or old, they seem to invite the doctors and nurses caring for them to change their roles from 'professional advisers and attendants' to intimate companions on the loneliest journey a human being ever takes.

Some years ago, I and a nursing colleague visited a woman at her doctor's request. She had advanced oesophageal carcinoma with considerable pain and almost total dysphagia. As is my custom, I did not immediately take a history, but rather asked the patient in what way she felt I could help her: 'Ease my pain, show me what I can eat, and reassure me that you will always answer my questions honestly. I must be fit enough to finish some unfinished business.'

Some weeks later, so frail that she could no longer manage at home, she was admitted to the hospice where, again, she was asked the same question: 'In what way can I be of service to you?' Surprisingly, she replied with a question: 'Do you know what a platform ticket is?' She proceeded to explain that she expected to meet a kindly companion in the near future. 'I feel as though I am on a railway platform, bags packed, a single ticket in my pocket and (just like British Rail!) my train is a trifle late. As if I had studied the travel brochures, I am excited about where I am going because it sounds so lovely but, of course, I haven't actually met anyone who has ever been there and I can't help feeling a bit apprehensive. As I wait here I would like someone to talk to, someone to advise me and possibly provide a bit of reassurance but, most of all, I just want a companion because I am finding it all a bit lonely. Will you get a platform ticket, doctor?'

It became a routine to stop at her bed and ask if it was time to buy the platform ticket, with always the same reply, 'No, so long as you know when to get it!' One day, scarcely looking any different, she called over and whispered that her train was coming in. I sat with her, holding her hand and marvelling that conversation seemed unnecessary, until she said 'Thank you for being with me—you can't come any further but I am no longer afraid or lonely,' and shortly afterwards she died.

That vignette says much from which we can learn, though admittedly she was exceptional in being so articulate (and colourful) as well as so trusting.

'TELLING' OR CONFIRMING

Doctors involved in the care of the dying are often surprised at how much many patients know about their diagnosis. Many have already been given information skilfully by colleagues, particularly if they are younger patients who must be able to give informed consent and willing co-operation for what, in the case of cancer patients, may be protracted regimens of surgery, radiotherapy, and chemotherapy. An equal number, however, have no recollection of being informed but have deduced the sinister prognosis from the changed attitude of their medical attendants, the altered pace of treatment, the whispered conversations outside the bedroom, the painful embarrassment of loved ones, and their ever-worsening physical health in spite of so much care and attention.

Rarely does the doctor find himself formally spelling out the diagnosis, but rather *confirming* the patient's suspicions, which often were aroused even before help was first sought. But the doctor is often expected to explain the cause and the significance of the symptoms—not because they are seen as diagnostic pointers, but as indicators of possible new problems or the source of fresh fears. Dysphagia is feared, not because it reminds the patient of the carcinoma he has discovered he harbours, but as a cause of choking or slow starvation. It is not so much the patient's bronchogenic carcinoma that needs an explanation, but whether the dyspnoea will lead to suffocation, or whether the copious sweating means he also has an infectious condition. He wants to know whether his 'muddledness' is normal or the herald of insanity; whether his weakness is the onset of paralysis; or whether the fleck of blood in the sputum is a forerunner of catastrophic haemorrhage.

He welcomes an invitation to speak of anything that troubles him, however trivial it may sound. He does not expect a new prescription for each symptom, but only some evidence of the doctor's genuine interest in how he feels. While the greeting 'How is the pain today?' may elicit an answer gratifying for the doctor who has controlled the pain effectively, the patient would usually much prefer to be asked 'How are *you* today?', so that he can speak about *anything* that is troubling him, even if the doctor seems inept at dealing with his concerns.

ACTIVE LISTENING

The doctor, with his fund of knowledge and ready answers, may find it disconcerting when he is expected to listen rather than expound, to be inactive when he would be more comfortable writing out a prescription or ordering further (often unnecessary) investigations. At all stages of his professional life he will be surprised at how often he is remembered as being 'helpful' or 'reassuring' when he recollects only sitting, listening, and perhaps feeling utterly helpless.

Few people are so conscious of taking up the time of others as those who have less of it remaining for themselves. Whereas the doctor may fear that caring for the dying 'will demand so much time', he is likely to find that the dying are not demanding, and as death approaches they ask less and less of their attendants and companions and are usually considerate to the point of embarrassment. It is as if they feel that the brevity of their remnant of life gives them no claim to the time and energies of another.

'HOW LONG, DOCTOR?'

Two aspects of this caring 'ministry' (for such it is) may frighten the most experienced doctor. The first is the way in which patients ask for a prognosis ('Though I know, of course, you can't give that, doctor') and then reinterpret whatever was said. 'Many weeks' is seen as less than eight because otherwise the doctor would surely have said 'two months'. 'Many, many months' may be interpreted as less than a year or even six months because it is thought that otherwise the doctor would have related it to (say) Christmas or the summer, and so on. Nothing, however, is more damaging and upsetting than giving a ridiculously vague prognosis such as 'two months to two years'. Invariably, the patient and family latch on to the more optimistic one and then wonder what has gone wrong and who is to blame when it turns out to be dramatically less favourable.

The other problem arises when questions of faith are raised, often thereby challenging the doctor to examine his own beliefs or philosophy, which, unlike the patient, he may not have even begun to formulate. His professional training may have taught him to regard this as such an intensely personal, private area of life as to be almost a taboo subject, and his relationship as one in which he must never been seen to proselytize or impose his views. On the other hand, since he is now regarded as a friend and companion, he should feel comfortable enough to let the patient express the whole range of emotions from anger to serenity, despair to hope. Sharing one's feelings about life, death, God, and love is right and proper within such a close and sensitive relationship.

The terminally ill patient principally seeks confirmation of what is happening and seems more concerned about the manner of his 'dying' than 'death' itself. Although he dwells more on the quality of his present life than on thoughts of the life to come, he may, by alluding to matters of faith or philosophy, embarrass the doctor, whom he now treats, perhaps without realizing it, more as a trusted confidant than a respected professional adviser.

So far, as will have become obvious, we have been describing somewhat unexpected reactions and questions that may surprise the doctor.

PROTECTING THE DOCTOR

The doctor is likely to be even more surprised when he realizes how much he is being protected by the patient. Not only is his busy professional and social life respected, but very often the patient engages in subtle deception as much for the sake of the doctor as for anyone else's. How often I have been called to see a patient by a colleague and asked the patient whether he knows and understands what is the matter with him, only to have the patient look around him to make sure no one can overhear and then say 'I am being treated for bronchitis but actually I have cancer! Promise me you won't tell my doctor I have found out—he has been so kind and considerate I would hate him to be hurt, or upset that I found out what he was trying to shield me from!' On other occasions, when a slight change in medication is being considered, the patient will say 'I hope my doctor won't feel I am not pleased with all he has done—I would never want to disappoint him.'

This same unselfish consideration for others usually extends to loved ones also. The patient who finds it both easy and helpful to chat with his doctor about every detail of his illness and what lies ahead may, right to his death, speak with his family as though he is as ignorant of it all as they had hoped and indeed worked for him to be.

I learned much from an occasion when a patient asked to speak to me and proceeded to go through a checklist of 22 questions ranging from how he would die to possible hymns for his funeral service! Suddenly, his wife's face appeared round his bedside curtains and, quick as a flash, his face broke into a smile as he said 'Oh darling, I wish you could have been here. Doctor has just been discussing cars with me and suggests that for our touring holiday in Spain next year we would be better with a new Metro!' Later the wife demanded to see me to upbraid me for daring to suggest that her husband (who died five days later) had any idea of how ill he was. Their mutual behaviour towards each other was, however, quite appropriate. He showed his love by protecting her, and his pragmatism by discussing every question that mattered to him with someone who could bear to help him. *She* was happy to think that she had shielded him as she must have done so often in their life together.

At other times, the growth of a human spirit approaching death may mystify relatives, or even hurt them, and here the doctor has a special role. Often the selfish man becomes unexpectedly considerate and generous; the shy person becomes more outgoing and confident; the critical or abrasive one becomes appreciative and gentle. This is not the effect of psychotropic drugs or the result of cerebral metastases, but the response of the human spirit that comes when someone is nursed in an atmosphere of love and support, free from bitterness, aggression, conflict, and destructive criticism. After a lifetime of domestic strife and mutual resentment this 'new person' image can be particularly hurtful for the one who is being left behind. 'How can he be so charming now after the way he has treated me for 30 years?'

PROTECTING THE RELATIVES

This leads us to look at another aspect of caring for the dying—caring for their relatives. A general practitioner will not need to be reminded that the immediate relatives are as much his concern as the patient is. Indeed, he may look forward to being their trusted doctor and friend for many years to come. In hospital, all attention seems to be focused on the patient, and hospital doctors tend to pay less attention to the needs of relatives than they merit, judging by studies carried out in a number of centres.

The needs of relatives are obviously different from those of the patient and may be skilfully concealed behind questions that seem to be entirely about the patient and his welfare. Through experince, it becomes clearer that much of their concern about the patient's suffering is not only a reflection of their love but also of their guilt (unjustified as it may be), their sense of failure or inadequacy, and their profound (and often quite justified) apprehension about their own future.

CARING FOR RELATIVES

The doctor who confines himself to speaking to relatives only about the patient, his investigations, treatment, prognosis, etc., and fails to ask '. . . and now tell me how *you* are getting on' is failing to understand the breadth of his professional role. A patient's improved appetite in hospital may be seen as an indication of his wife's culinary inadequacy at home. His relaxed mood may be construed as the result of his being taken out of her anxious care, or his persisting pain and discomfort as due to her nursing incompetence.

Similar examples abound. For the patient, death is the end of suffering, possibly (if he is blessed with a faith) the promise of better things to come. For the relative, death is only the beginning of a chapter of life so different, so daunting, that he or she can scarcely bear to look into the future.

Nothing could be more important for patient or relative (for their delicately interwoven reactions influence symptoms and prognosis) than for the doctor *always* to set time aside for the *personal, particular needs* of the relatives. The one who is to be left must be invited and encouraged to express how he or she really feels. To the doctor's surprise, a wife may describe how relieved she is to know that her husband's death is imminent because that will signal the end of his suffering *or* the chance for her of a new life that can only be better than the one she has endured for many years. She may just want to say how uncomfortable it is to sit by the bedside or how upsetting it it is to see him so changed for better or worse. She may want to be reassured that someone will visit and support her after the death during the months and years that will bring loneliness and a sense of 'aloneness' she had never known before. While the patient may regain a faith, so the relatives may lose faith and find it replaced with bitterness and anger, often directed at the medical profession or even God himself. Relatives, every bit as much as patients, need to be given encouragement and permission to 'be themselves', to express their true feelings, whether tearful, angry, relieved, or fearful, and to be accepted as they are.

A widow once remarked to me that she wished I could be as good with relatives as I had been with the patient, her late husband. 'I used to feel so angry with you when you came downstairs each day, put an arm om my shoulder, and told me how well I was caring for him. You never once asked me how I *really* felt, about how angry I was, how frightened, how let down!' Such conversations with relatives about their personal feelings must, obviously, be confidential, but this need not prevent the doctor telling the patient that he is meeting with the relatives to try to help them too, provided that at all times he reassures the patient that there are no secrets being withheld from him.

At the heart of all 'talking with the dying' must be complete honesty and openness, founded on professional skill, competence, and empathy. Only a foolish doctor believes he must appear omnipotent! His patients, and particularly those who are dying and their families, are likely to recognize his frailities, but usually respect him all the more for them if, in every single encounter, he remains a friend who can express humanity, humility, and humour.

18 Talking about pregnancy and reproduction

Normal pregnancy is not an illness, and so the mother to be rightly assumes a much less dependent role. The attendants' central concern should be to stimulate confidence and self-reliance in preparation for motherhood. Child-bearing is thus likely to be experienced as a challenge, putting the woman on her mettle. But some of the vocabulary often used by professionals can be insensitive, so that, by their choice of words, they not only filch for themselves much of the credit for the woman's achievement—by 'supervising' her pregnancy, 'managing' her labour, and 'delivering' the infant—but in some cases may appear to stigmatize the mother through the use of terms that could imply inadequacy. The 'growth retarded' infant has a 'poor' score on biophysical profile; a failed induction or failure to progress then necessitates operative intervention. Bastian [109] drew attention to the way in which this sort of terminology can erode the self-confidence that sensitive care would seek to foster.

THE 'HAPPY EVENT'

It is important to understand the range of attitudes and reactions to pregnancy which may be encountered. While we refer elsewhere (p. 219) to the value which human societies traditionally attach to fertility, nevertheless, a conception which for one couple may cause unalloyed delight may represent for another woman economic disaster through the loss of her job, or her prospects of a career; while for a third woman the pregnancy may be an absolute personal catastrophe.

Mixed and shifting feelings, too, are common as the woman sometimes struggles to weigh up the positive and negative consequences which the pregnancy may bring in its train. It is prudent, therefore, not to rush automatically into conventional congratulations: 'I've good news for you, you're pregnant!', but to tune in carefully to what the woman is feeling, 'What are your plans if the test is positive?', 'How do you feel now your pregnancy has been confirmed?'

AN EDUCATIONAL OPPORTUNITY

Pregnancy is typically a time of special health consciousness. It therefore usually affords a unique opportunity, over a period of several months, for closer communication between the woman and her attendant(s), sharing the same objective of a successful pregnancy with a healthy baby. The relationship is less liable to be clouded by the anxiety which often attends illness. The expectant mother's openness to advice provides opportunities for many aspects of health to be addressed, such as diet and nutrition; hygiene and prevention of infection; immunization; smoking, alcohol, drugs affecting health; anatomy and physiology of reproduction; conception and family planning.

Whatever the mother-to-be learns about health, she is likely to teach by example and precept to her family, so that the initial educational message is amplified. Consistency of advice avoids confusion and loss of confidence.

HIGHER EXPECTATIONS: GREATER PRESSURE TO GET IT RIGHT

As pregnancy outcome has improved over the years, women's expectations have risen and most women assume that their pregnancy will end successfully. This only highlights the sense of uncertainty and inadequacy often felt by the woman whose previous pregnancy was unsuccessful. Commonly, she may not dare to invest any positive feelings in the pregnancy until some time after the child is born, and she may be too ashamed to voice her lack of confidence, and her inability to indulge in the happiness which others expect her to be feeling. Similar feelings may be experienced by the woman whose current pregnancy is complicated by bleeding, growth retardation, or some other potentially ominous condition.

NORMAL PREGNANCY

Two trends in contemporary obstetric practice have considerable implications for communication. First, at the same time that the focus of medical concern has shifted from controlling maternal mortality to minimizing perinatal loss, 'access' to the unborn infant (through new technologies) has opened up dramatically. As a consequence, in the antenatal clinic it is the development, growth, and well-being of the unborn infant that is the centre of medical interest and concern, often more than the condition of the mother. *Her* observations and concerns can easily be overlooked or pushed to one side. She may begin to feel more like a mere baby receptacle than a person!

Second, the amount of information now gathered by tests of various sorts during the course of each pregnancy has expanded enormously. This implies a correspondingly greater need to communicate to the mother the significance of these many additional items of information about her pregnancy. To offer just one simple but symbolic example, the ultrasound scanning screen needs to be angled so that the mother as well as the doctor can see and understand what is happening to her baby.

Talking with a woman during her pregnancy embraces several themes. These include the following:

- health education (as already discussed);

- listening to the woman's concerns, interpreting for her the subjective experiences of pregnancy, reassuring her about minor deviations from 'normal';

- promoting self-confidence and self-reliance in preparation for motherhood;

- explaining the significance of tests, scans, screening procedures, other observations, and answering questions;

- discussing options, especially if any intervention is in prospect.

Labour and delivery

As the time for labour approaches, fear of a painful ordeal is by no means always the woman's major concern. Her thoughts are more likely to dwell on other practical issues, such as:

- Will the baby be normal and well?

- How will she react to the pain and stress of labour? Will she lose control or let herself down? Will she be able to co-operate with the midwife well enough to avoid medical intervention?

- Will she be spared a genital shave?

- What pain relief will she be offered?

- Will she be able to move about and choose her own positions in labour?

- Can her husband remain with her throughout?

- Who will be present at her delivery, and who will actually deliver her? Will she require stitches?

- How will her toddler cope with the separation while she is in hospital?

This list is not exhaustive. It is always helpful to encourage the woman to spell out beforehand the questions in her mind, and then to provide her with clear answers. These can be recorded in her case folder as a birth plan, which will communicate her wishes to all the staff who will attend her in labour.

Puerperium

During the postnatal period, as the woman returns to her everyday domestic activities, the primipara is taking on for the first time the complex, demanding challenge of motherhood; the multipara has added to her multifarious responsibilities. It is, not surprisingly, a stressful period, when the mother may lose her self-confidence and become depressed, and this is commonly overlooked. Occasionally, couples who cannot cope will begin to neglect or physically abuse their infant.

Various health professionals are usually around to guide and support the woman during this time—health visitors, clinic or hospital staff, the family doctor, not to mention mothers and mothers-in-law! But if she receives conflicting advice from different sources, as readily happens, she may become confused and lose confidence. The family doctor is often in the best position to ensure liaison among the various givers of advice, and to co-ordinate their efforts. For an extended period after birth, women are likely to consult their general practitioner with increased frequency. The mother requires special support where the baby is adopted, fostered, or taken into care, or when it remains for a long time in a special care baby unit.

PREGNANCY LOSS: ABORTION OR PERINATAL DEATH

Most unsuccessful pregnancies end in the very earliest weeks, after a defective embryo has died. These losses can be represented as Nature's quality control at work—as pregnancies that were never meant to continue. Most, again, are random events, and not the expression of some continuing genetic defect.

Doctors and nurses are therefore inclined to dismiss a miscarriage as an event of no great significance, something that is 'all for the best'. But for the couple concerned it may be experienced as a bereavement (see also p.78) and the woman's feelings of grief, loss, and failure are more deeply felt when the miscarriage has followed a period of infertility. The woman's distress will also be compounded if her doctor seems to trivialize the miscarriage, and treats it as a commonplace event of no great medical significance.

Often the woman feels blameworthy. Was it due to something she did, or did not do, she asks herself. She is likely to scan her family tree, looking for any evidence of a reproductive taint, and may attach significance to quite unrelated events. Her concern is greatly intensified if miscarriage is recurrent. The sense of loss may not be oppressive immediately, but may develop later, possibly around the anniversary of a miscarriage or still birth. The loss of one of twins leads to confused feelings of grief and happiness, which the parents may find difficulty in expressing.

INFERTILITY

Infertile couples are often not handled well by their doctors, who are inclined to make light of their concern and to brush aside their anxieties. This may be in part because the doctor has not personally experienced their predicament; because infertility may not be seen as a true 'medical' problem; and because a significant proportion of infertility is either inexplicable or irremediable, and therefore baffles the doctor. One needs only to look around the faces of those waiting in an infertility clinic to recognize the feelings of inadequacy and even shame which they commonly reflect.

On most occasions, an infertile couple should be seen together. They should be given opportunities to voice their anxiety and other unhappy feelings, and to acknowledge any strains within their relationship, general or sexual. When investigation points to the need to consider some form of assisted reproduction (such as artificial insemination by husband or donor, *in vitro* fertilization, or GIFT, or to contemplate adoption, a counselling approach is desirable. In this way one can make available the breadth of information, support, and guidance which is required for making decisions in this special situation. The couple are liable to feel inadequate, or guilty and blameworthy.

Throughout their care, there will be repeated opportunities for health education in many aspects of the anatomy and physiology of reproduction. Line drawings, wallcharts, and booklets are very useful in this regard.

FAMILY PLANNING

Doctors can feel reluctant to talk with patients about family planning for a variety of reasons:

- They may imagine that some criticism of the patient could be inferred. 'Why did she become pregnant again in her present circumstances?'; 'Why has she allowed such a short interval between her babies?'

- They may be afraid of appearing anti-natalist especially with patients from pro-natalist cultures, who have a very different notion of desired family size.

- They may feel that so personal a topic should be first raised by the patient, rather than the doctor.

- They may feel uncomfortable if the patient is not married.

However, it should always be possible to discuss this important aspect of health in an acceptable way without appearing intrusive. If the patient's knowledge of, attitudes to, and experience of contraception are not known, the time-course of her reproductive history can often provide an entrée:

'When do you hope to start/add to your family?' 'Was it from choice or necessity that you waited *x* years before adding to your family?' 'Did you plan to have this baby quite soon after the previous birth?'

Patients' responses to questions such as these will usually give some initial indication of their contraceptive experience, if any.

It is then important to obtain in more detail a contraceptive history. What particular methods have the couple tried, considered, or discarded? What side-effects, anxieties, misapprehensions, or other concerns have influenced their choices? Have they already found a mutually satisfactory method?

This information needs to be elicited in a non-judgemental way, without any implication that (say) the patient's lack of knowledge means that she is dim or irresponsible, or that her fears and misconceived ideas about particular methods mean that she is foolish and immature. The motivation to persist with a particular method is only likely to be sustained if the choice is indeed the patient's own, and not just something which the doctor thinks would be good for her.

Talking about contraception again provides repeated opportunities to inform and educate patients regarding the anatomy and physiology of reproduction, and to introduce them to suitable vocabulary to describe sexual function.

Sterilization

Although a spouse's consent is not legally required before sterilization is performed in Britain, it is wise to find out his or her attitude. Normally the best practice is to talk to the couple together, so that they can jointly confirm that their family is complete, and each of them can express their views and concerns. The couple should understand that sterilization is planned to produce permanent conception control, but this should never be cast up reproachfully at the patient returning later in changed circumstances with a request for attempted reversal. The procedure is unlikely to lead to future regret provided it follows a settled decision, best reached away from the time of recent delivery or abortion.

TERMINATION OF PREGNANCY

When a woman seeks advice and help regarding termination of her pregnancy, in conformity with the abortion laws in Britain the doctor must be willing to certify that continuance of the pregnancy would be a greater threat than abortion to the patient's physical or mental health. In making this assessment, particularly in relation to the woman's mental health, a central issue is 'What does the patient truly want for herself?' It is not unusual for the woman to have ambivalent feelings, so that she may appear confused and susceptible to pressure from any direction. In seeking to arrive at a settled decision, therefore, it is important to discover whether the woman is exposed to external pressures—from her partner, her family, or other sources.

The woman herself, or the doctor, may have ethical reservations about the circumstances in which abortion is justified. When this is so, these issues are best brought into the open, and honestly acknowledged.

The doctor needs to ensure that she knows about the methods to be used; that she understands the alternatives, and the likely outcome of particular procedures. Although delay must be avoided, it can sometimes be helpful to arrange a second interview within a few days if there is uncertainty about the wisest course of action.

Despite feeling great relief in the short-term, few women escape a sense of loss following termination of pregnancy, sometimes tinged with regret or guilt. [110] Follow-up interviews, which can help to work through these feelings, are often not well attended in a hospital clinic. They therefore tend to become the responsibility of the family doctor.

Talking about sexual function

The need for doctors to desexualize the intimacy of clinical work has been identified in earlier chapters as a factor that inhibits them from discussing patients' sexual function, or even other 'personal' matters. Nevertheless, with insight and training this reluctance can and should be overcome, since health problems related to sexual function are not rarities. Surveys in general practice have shown that 10–15 per cent of patients have a sexual problem of some sort. Sexual problems apart, enquiry about contraceptive practice is often an appropriate part of history-taking. The widespread prevalence of sexually transmitted diseases means that doctors in all specialties have to keep these infections in mind in dealing with disorders of many body systems, and to be informed about the pattern of the patient's sexual behaviour.

However, enquires about a patient's sexual function need not form a part of routine history-taking. First, the doctor has to consider carefully the nature of the patient's presenting symptoms, their possible causes, and likely consequences. Enquiry would certainly be appropriate when a patient's physical condition or current medication could affect normal sexual function, or when the presenting complaint is vague ('feeling run down', 'being out of sorts', 'not feeling my normal self'), without obvious explanation, or when there are other indications of unexplained anxiety or depression.

As in other areas of medicine, it is helpful to keep in mind the epidemiology of the disorder i.e. the circumstances in which the prevalence of sexual difficulty is likely to be greater and when, therefore, enquiry would be appropriate. These include situations such as:

- the patient first seeking contraceptive advice;

- the patient presenting with symptoms of possible sexually transmitted disease;

- the woman presenting with her first pregnancy;

- the woman appearing for postnatal examination;

- the patient who has undergone surgical mutilation, e.g. mastectomy, a bowel stoma, an amputation;

- the woman with a gynaecological complaint, particularly one causing genital pain or tenderness;

- the patient with a disorder likely to result in sexual dysfunction, e.g. diabetes, alcohol abuse, multiple sclerosis, severe arthritis;

- the patient receiving medication that can affect sexual function, e.g. some hypotensive drugs, psychotropics, diuretics;

- the patient, male or female, experiencing climacteric symptoms;

- the patient who indicates that there are problems in the marital relationship.

HOW TO INTRODUCE THE TOPIC

Broaching the topic of sexual function during history-taking calls for delicacy combined with directness. Timing is important, and rapport with the patient should first be established. The questions asked should be unambiguous, and should convey by their openness the doctor's comfort with the topic and readiness to talk. The vocabulary chosen should consist of words that the patient is likely to understand, not too formally 'medical', nor slangy or vulgar.

The pattern of enquiry depends on whether the patient has acknowledged the existence of a sexual problem, or whether the doctor has decided to take the initiative in raising the topic because he believed it to be relevant to the patient's complaints. Considering the latter situation first: if the patient is married, a suitable simple direct question would be 'Are you able to enjoy sexual intercourse comfortably?' In the case of an older person, the question could be modified 'Are you still able to enjoy sexual intercourse comfortably?' If the patient answers affirmatively to such an enquiry, usually no more questions need be asked.

Questions in these terms do not imply that a sexual problem exists, and are therefore likely to be received better than the enquiry 'Do you have a sexual problem?'

When the patient is single and the doctor does not know whether a sexual relationship exists or not, it may appear best to enquire about boyfriends or girlfriends before asking 'Are you having a sexual relationship?' Alternatively, and perhaps preferably, a simple direct approach can again be adopted. A useful question from which to begin, particularly with a young teenager, would be 'Have you ever had sexual intercourse?' This takes account of the tentative and sporadic nature of much sexual activity in the teenage years. If the answer is 'Yes', then 'Have you a partner now?' is appropriate, followed by the same sort of question described for a married person, 'Are you able to enjoy sexual intercourse comfortably?'

When the patient is ostensibly without a partner—divorced, widowed, or separated—particular tact is required. In the case of a widow or widower, the doctor may prefer first to ask tentatively 'How do you cope with your sexual feelings since you lost your partner?' But again it may be more fitting to ask directly 'Have you met a new sexual partner since you were divorced/separated/widowed?' If the doctor is unsure about the patient's sexual orientation, he can ask directly 'Are you attracted sexually to women, or men, or both?'

Turning to the situation in which the patient has indicated that a sexual problem exists, sometimes the complaint is vague or unspecified 'Well, to be honest, doctor, I want to talk to you about my sex life. It's a disaster area!' 'Actually, doctor, I've lost all interest in married life.' 'I guess I'm not much use to my wife nowadays.' It can then be helpful to explore the difficulty initially with one or two more general questions about the patient's subjective experience, such as:

'Do you look forward to making love?'
'Do you get aroused/turned on?'
'Does love-making make you feel happy and relaxed?'
'Do you find intercourse uncomfortable or painful?'

Questions of this sort, in opening up the topic, allow patients to talk first about their general sexual feelings and responses. Then it is appropriate to find out what specific difficulties occur. If the patient has not already given an indication of what is going wrong, the questions should cover the main aspects of sexual response. For a woman, does good lubrication occur with arousal, does she get wet enough? Is satisfaction (climax) usually attained? For a man, is there difficulty in getting or keeping an erection? Does the man come (ejaculate) too quickly?

Once a clearer picture of the difficulties has been obtained, the doctor should find out when and how the problem started. It is often useful to go back to the start of the relationship. Was there difficulty then, and if not, when did the problem develop? Were there any concurrent events that might have led to the problem, e.g. illness, loss of a job, strain in the relationship, infidelity, bereavement? It is usually appropriate to ask at some point in the history how often the couple make love and, if intercourse is infrequent, when the last time was. More general questions are then called for about the couple's opportunities for affectionate interaction. Do they go out and about much together? Do they display affection outside the bedroom? Do they usually retire to bed together? Who usually makes the first move? Does the couple share any physical affection that is not just a preliminary to coitus?

When sexual unresponsiveness is part of the problem, the patient can be asked whether feelings of sexual interest occur when the partner is not present or when intercourse is not in prospect.

To have a better understanding of the patient's current difficulties, it is often helpful to discover more about attitudes to sexuality acquired during childhood, and about the earliest sexual experiences:

- What sex education did the patient receive as a child?

- Were sexual matters something that could be discussed in the home?

- What warnings or prohibitions did the patient receive as a child?

- Was the patient as a child fondled or otherwise sexually exploited by an adult, particularly a member of the family?

- Did any sexually alarming episodes occur during childhood or adolescence?

Regarding early sexual experience, it might be seen as accusatory to ask 'Was your husband/wife, fiancé(e) the first person you ever made love to?' A better question is 'Can you remember your very first sexual experience? When did that happen?' From this beginning it will be possible to trace the patient's sexual relationship(s), and to discover whether difficulties similar to the current ones were present earlier.

If the doctor has had no special training or experience in helping patients with sexual problems, he may feel that, having identified the problem, the best course is to refer the patient to someone with appropriate skills. If, however, he decides to find out more about the problem, the sort of information required can be summarized under the following headings.

Erectile impotence

This can be due to organic or functional causes, and appropriate questions should provide a pointer. Do normal erections occur on waking from dreaming sleep, and during fantasy and masturbation? If the impotence is limited to situations where intercourse is attempted or is in prospect, is an erection achieved and then lost, or is there complete erectile failure? When the condition is secondary (i.e. preceded by normal erectile function), it is important to know whether the onset was gradual or abrupt.

Premature ejaculation

Establish whether ejaculation occurs before complete erection, before penetration, or shortly thereafter. Is it controlled more easily during masturbation? After ejaculating once, can the man become aroused again and continue for longer before ejaculating on the second occasion?

Failure to ejaculate

These cases are by no means rare, and may present as unexplained infertility. One should find out whether the difficulty is situational, i.e. whether it is only within the vagina that the patient has difficulty in ejaculating. Is there a history of practising coitus interruptus or reservatus during early sexual experience?

In female patients, the most common problem is some form of *sexual unresponsiveness*, usually secondary. It is important to distinguish between lack of sexual interest or appetite (the woman who never thinks or feels 'sexy'); impaired responsiveness (the woman who feels interest, but fails to respond during love-making); and orgasmic difficulty (failure to climax). It is helpful to enquire whether the patient is more responsive to manual caresses than to vaginal coitus. Can she experience arousal by masturbating? Do her difficulties relate only to her present partner? Does her partner spend enough time in foreplay? Is he rough, indifferent, or demanding? Does he ejaculate too quickly?

Vaginismus

These cases are likely to present as failure to consummate a marriage (sometimes after many years) or as unexplained infertility. Can the patient allow anything to enter her vagina? Her own finger? Her partner's finger? A tampon? Did she experience alarming episodes or admonitions in childhood? Can she experience satisfactory arousal if penetration is not attempted?

Most patients with sexual problems are quite ready to talk about them to a doctor who shows concern, understanding, and, perhaps most importantly, comfort with the topic. As the doctor learns the appropriate way to phrase his questions, he will be surprised to discover how easy it is to include this important aspect of health in his history-taking.

Talking about sexually transmitted diseases (Including HIV infection)

For many doctors and other health workers, it is particularly difficult to talk with patients about this aspect of health, because of the uncomfortable feelings which the topic is liable to evoke. On the patient's side, there is likely to be embarrassment, but there may also be guilt, outraged innocence, or indifferent bravado. Feelings apart, the patient may lack the vocabulary needed to give an adequate account of the history.

There is a special need, therefore, for the doctor to gain the patient's confidence by demonstrating his acceptance (p. 62); by avoiding judgemental language or behaviour; and by emphasizing the confidentiality of the consultation.

The doctor may sometimes find it difficult to maintain a proper and professional objectivity because of the intrusion of his personal

attitudes and values. The frailties of human sexual behaviour sometimes glimpsed as the history unfolds—irresponsibility, betrayal of
trust, selfishness—may tempt the doctor to take a judgemental
stance. In this way his ability to help the patient personally can
quickly be destroyed, and the mutual trust needed for effective
tracing of contacts will evaporate.

Rather than indulging in sexual moralizing, the doctor must
remind himself of the extent to which health problems generally
are the self-imposed consequences of flawed human behaviour. If
we exclude for the moment genetically determined disorders and
iatrogenic illnesses, a very high proportion of the remaining burden
of ill health in the developed world is self-induced, from road
traffic injuries through smoking-related disorders, ill health due
to obesity, alcohol-induced illness, other drug abuse problems—
the list is endless!

Infection with the human immunodeficiency virus (HIV), usually sexually transmitted, is currently spreading on a pandemic
scale. It is unique in its uncertain course, but probably lethal
outcome. The AIDS syndrome which results from infection is
surrounded by fear and much ignorance, despite public health
information campaigns. The risk of infection has already had some
influence on patterns of sexual behaviour, and attitudes to casual
sexual contacts.

Although free, confidential blood testing for HIV is available
in Britain, some individuals may be reluctant to undergo a test,
because of the inferences which may be drawn by insurance
companies and other agencies, even when the test in negative,
and because of fear of the repercussions of a positive test on
that individual's whole way of life. These are likely to involve
not just his future health, but his social and sexual relationships
and possibly his employment. For a woman, the risk of vertical
transmission of the virus to an unborn child is liable to cast a dark
cloud of fear over her reproductive future.

For these reasons, it is prudent that those seeking testing
should, before testing as well as when a result is obtained, be
counselled by someone knowledgeable about the natural history
of HIV infection, and its personal implications for the patient.
Those individuals who feel the need for greater anonymity can
get information and advice from AIDS telephone helplines.

People need clear advice about how they can avoid infection, or avoid transmitting it to others, so the doctor must be ready to talk explicitly and comfortably about the potential risks of different forms of sexual intimacy.

Patients carrying the human immunodeficiency virus (and/or other blood-borne viruses such as hepatitis B and C) may evoke alarm or even rejection from staff when they are admitted to hospital, because of the fear of cross-transmission of the virus. Untested patients from high-risk groups may set off similar reactions, particularly in surgical units. The risk to staff of cross-infection can be contained only be adopting standard precautions to avoid contact with blood or infective secretions. But this should not lead on to the social isolation of the patient, and the withdrawal of all physical contacts. On the contrary, there is a need to compensate for the inevitable effects of the measures taken to avoid contagion, by using touch contact and other demonstrations of acceptance.

As patients develop the full-blown AIDS syndrome, they face an inexorable decline in their condition. They present a growing challenge to those providing health care, not only in terms of resources, but in providing the support and true caring needed as they try to come to terms with their plight.

20 Aspects of transcultural communication

With travellers, visitors, and immigrants from many countries of the world very much part of the everyday scene, doctors need to broaden their understanding of how best to communicate with patients from other cultures, avoiding the difficulties that can arise through ignorance of their customs and beliefs.

In a short chapter, there is a risk of seeming to sketch stereotypes. This I have tried to avoid, but it is only possible to attempt very incomplete outlines of certain general cultural patterns.

GREETINGS

The formalities of greeting are often more prolonged among non-Europeans. While a handshake has become pretty universal, it is something many Indian women avoid. Use of a given (first) name alone is a familiarity in Britain, but is normal in the Islamic world, even in formal situations. In Japanese culture, surnames are usual.

BODY LANGUAGE

Head-shaking signifying refusal in Britain indicates assent in South Asian countries. In Japan and China, every effort is made to mask any show of emotion, to avoid inflicting it on others: so grief or anger are concealed with an (apparently inappropriate) smile. Uninhibited laughter is considered bad manners in Southern Asia, but is commonplace among Africans. In many African and South Asian cultures, it is good manners to avoid direct eye contact with a superior—which the doctor is likely to be seen as. The resulting downcast gaze may be misinterpreted as evidence of unreliability, or withdrawal and depression.

LANGUAGE

Some languages are more precise and explicit than others, which have an inherent vagueness. But apart from these linguistic differences, there are also important cultural differences in the way language is used. In Britain (and northern Europe generally) information is conveyed by words clearly spelt out. In much of the rest of the world, meaning and understanding rely much more on non-verbal communication—pauses, silences, body language, the context of the words—rather than on explicit statements.

In the Japanese tradition, there is a clear distinction between one's public posture, and personal feelings. The underlying truth, which is rarely articulated, has to be divined by subtle guesswork. In Japan, doctors habitually collude with relatives in concealing the diagnosis of cancer—an expression of the need to avoid evoking or displaying emotions painful to another.

Unless the patient is fluent in English, it is helpful to speak slowly, spacing the words a little, and throwing in synonyms to make the meaning clearer. Use familiar words, not slang, colloquialisms, or technical jargon. Sometimes use of a proverb may help to reinforce a point—'We have a saying "A stitch in time saves nine." Is there a similar saying in your language? There is! Good! That is what I am trying to explain to you!'

If patient and doctor do not have a common language, they may have to communicate through an interpreter. A relative, a trusted friend, or even a stranger of the same sex as the patient can fulfil this role. Sometimes a teenage child of the family who has been educated in Britain may be the person in the family with the best command of English. Many hospitals have a panel of volunteer interpreters covering a wide range of languages. The presence of another person who is merely an interpreter may seriously inhibit the patient from disclosing 'personal' matters. On the other hand, a patient from another culture, perhaps feeling overawed or misunderstood, may wish for the company of a trusted friend or relative to assist communication, not merely as a translator, but as an advocate, to communicate the patient's perception of his illness.

Vocabulary, nevertheless, can present problems. There may be lack of appropriate corresponding words to describe both physical and emotional symptoms, and changes of mood. Even during interviews with native English-speaking patients, terms used either by the patient or by the doctor may be confusing and ambiguous and readily give rise to serious misconceptions. Examples of this sort of difficulty (from the field of neurology) were given by Hawkes [111]. Terms such as weakness, numbness, giddy or dizzy turns, neuritis, or migraine, for example, are liable to be used by doctors and patient without a clear mutual understanding of what the term is supposed to mean. These difficulties are much more likely to arise when the patient is from a different culture and speaks a different language.

Besides this, the patient's perception of his complaint and interpretation of the nature of his illness are likely to be much influenced by cultural frames of reference. For example, feeling unwell may be construed as a consequence of such diverse influences as astrological fate, impiety, a curse or spell, or even 'possession' by a spirit. These varying notions have a profound influence on the manner in which the complaint is perceived and described. Even within the confines of the Western world the same symptoms might be ascribed by a food faddist to an allergy to toxic additives, by a Christian Scientist to wrong thinking, or by an osteopath to vertebral derangement! Each would advocate a form of therapy appropriate to his notions of causality.

The language of distress adopted in different cultures to describe pain and illness may be emotional and dramatic (as in some Mediterranean cultures) creating an impression of neuroticism; or stoical and nonchalant (especially desert-dwellers and nomads, for whom endurance and handship are common place, possibly leading to under-investigation or dismissal; or it may be oblique: vague lower abdominal pain in women, or vague menstrual complaints, are in African and Arab cultures often the *cris de coeur* of the infertile woman.

A full review of culture-bound syndromes of illness-behaviour has been prepared by Littlewood and Lipsedge [112].

INFLUENCE OF FAMILY STRUCTURE
AND RELATIONSHIPS

Among the strongest elements of cultural influence are those
bound up with the pattern of everyday family living. In many
traditional cultures, particularly in rural settings, the family is
a compound group of members, with several generations living
together, and with young wives joining the family on marriage.

The head of the family

In most of these compound families, the senior male is regarded
as very much the head, whatever the influence the older women
customarily exercise backstage, in the privacy of the domestic
circle! The approval of the male head of the family may therefore
be considered necessary not only for major interventions such
as an operation, but for any decision about the medical care
of any member of the family. Further, it may be helpful when
a consultation takes place to involve the head of the family
whenever possible in the exposition, since compliance is likely to
depend crucially on his endorsement and reiteration of the doctor's
instructions.

The roles and attitudes of women

Where traditional cultures are still strong, the social roles of women
are very much centred in the domestic world—home-making, the
preparation of food, child-bearing and child-rearing. In rural
communities, these functions are often combined with many of
the most laborious family tasks, such as growing food, carrying
water, and gathering fuel.

In conservative Islamic cultures, women may be expected to
seclude themselves in the harem (*zenana*), the women's quarters
of the home. When they venture outside the home, 'respectable'
women avoid social (and certainly physical) contact with strangers,
and may practise veiling to a greater or lesser extent, depending
on the degree of conservatism in their community. In orthodox
Hindu communities also, women seek, wherever possible, to avoid
contact with others, particularly those of a lower caste.

These cultural patterns and attitudes exercise an important influence on many aspects of the lives of the women concerned. Females are likely to have received fewer years of schooling, to be less literate, and less able to speak English, so that verbal and written communication can be much more difficult. Of the estimated one billion adult illiterates world-wide, three-quarters are Asian and the majority are women. Such women, therefore, usually seek advice and information about aspects of their personal lives, including health matters, from older women, generally within the family, rather than from books, magazines, the media, and professional sources. Conversely, those women who do find themselves 'isolated' in a nuclear family may feel insecure, unsupported, and less able to make decisions for themselves. Young primiparae may be especially diffident about the care of the baby, if their mother or mother-in-law is not around to guide them.

A married woman's social standing is mainly derived from her reputation for 'respectability', i.e. conformity to the conventions of the culture, from the number of her children (particularly her sons), and from her seniority within the family group. In many parts of Africa and South Asia, a woman must deliver vaginally (not by Caesarean section) to maintain respect.

An unmarried female's good standing in southern Asian cultures is crucially dependent on her reputation for chaste behaviour—the assurance of her virginity. Women's need to protect their personal reputations throughout their lives has an influence not only on their general social behaviour but also on their attitudes towards clinical examination, with the undressing and exposure that inevitably occurs. Muslim women are taught the boundaries of the 'awra'—those areas of the body which must remain covered. A Hindu woman might cover her face with the hem of her sari during abdominal palpation, and is liable to adopt an expression of rather exaggerated distaste during vaginal examination, to emphasize her respectability and her aversion to the intimate contact with a person other than her husband. Many traditional women agree to clinical examination only if it is performed by a female doctor, with the husband's consent, or in his presence. Parents will often refuse to allow vaginal examination of an unmarried daughter.

The exclusiveness and privacy that characterize a couple's physical relationship in marriage makes it difficult for either of them to discuss this aspect of their lives, even with a doctor of the same sex. In an arranged marriage the wife in particular may have quite modest expectations of sexual fulfilment and she is for that reason less likely to sense that a sexual problem exists; and even if she does, she may well not think it seemly for a wife to voice such concerns.

The compound family

Relationships within the compound family are generally dominated by the hierarchy of age, the younger members regularly deferring to their elders. Even a small difference of age between siblings implies a corresponding ranking, and an obligation to defer. The senior, older members of the family almost automatically attract respect and prestige; women too, beyond the menopause, not only gain respect but often enjoy greater social freedom. But among orthodox Hindus, the remarriage of widows is not approved. The increasing dependence of the elderly and their idiosyncracies are accepted; and the responsibility for their care is usually shouldered without hesitation. Indeed, the proposal that an elderly relative be removed to hospital may be construed as a reflection upon the caring of the other family members, and therefore resisted. When a member of the family, of whatever age, is admitted to hospital, one or more of the relatives may well insist on remaining close by as an attendant. This exemplifies the sense of collective responsibility and mutual obligation within the compound family, even when all the members do not live under the same roof. Important decisions are usually made only after consultation within the family group.

The corollary of the respect accorded to the elderly is the submission and conformity expected of the young, and of the adolescent in particular. If this is not forthcoming, as is more likely to happen in an established immigrant family whose children have received all their education in Britain, great tension or even serious rifts can arise between the generations. These may centre on disagreements about conventional dressing, about choice of friends, or about social mixing with the opposite sex, but become more serious when the parents are planning an arranged marriage for their son or daughter who wishes to find his or her own partner.

Attempts at suicide are more common among Asian adolescent girls. This is only one instance of the special stresses which immigrants experience, living in an alien culture. Among

Caribbean immigrants, schizophrenic breakdown is more common.

Children

Throughout history, children have been seen as a family's great asset, a blessing from God. In communities dependent on peasant agriculture, children's contribution to the labour force is invaluable, especially during labour-intensive periods such as harvest. Sons in particular endow the family with greater financial security, with physical security (for the women, the land, the home) and with social security as the parents grow older. In Hindu culture, a son also affords spiritual security, through his important role in the funeral rites of his parents. Often, therefore, the birth of a daughter or, worse, another daughter, is liable to be greeted with muted joy or tears of disappointment.

But, for countless generations past, families have experienced the relentless toll of heavy infant and child mortality. Commonly, almost a half of those born have failed to survive to reach adolescence. A woman might expect only two surviving sons after bearing seven or eight children. As a consequence, in traditional cultures, pregnancy is celebrated, and children are welcomed, cossetted, and spoiled by their grandparents. Large families are idealized. Fertility is greatly valued, and infertility is regarded as the ultimate disaster.

High maternal mortality has also been an 'accepted' part of human experience from earliest times, and in many parts of the world high maternal mortality persists [113]. In those communities in which maternal mortality was high and fertility was uncontrolled, the life expectancy of women was strikingly *less* than that of men, in contrast to the longevity of women in the contemporary developed world. This experience must also have played an important part in shaping cultural attitudes to favour early marriage and high fertility. Unless a woman married early and bred frequently throughout her short life, the family might be in danger of extinction.

These deep-seated cultural values, often enshrined in religion, engender suspicion and hostility towards the control of fertility: towards contraception, sterilization, or abortion. Similarly, women refuse to consider hysterectomy, however severe their gynaecological problems. It is only when the survival of children can be demonstrated and assured that couples become willing to discuss contraception, and to contemplate restricting the size of their family.

The precarious nature of a young child's hold on life is acknowledged in a number of customs in different communities. The infant's hair may not be cut for many months, to avoid weakening it in any way. In the Indian and Arab tradition, dark powder (*kohl, surma*) is applied round the child's eyes, to 'protect' the child from illness. This powder sometimes contains lead or antimony compounds, which may poison the child. In some cultures, the child's naming ceremony is deferred for some considerable time after its birth to conceal, as it were, the child's existence and identity from malevolent influences. In the Arab tradition, a child should not be admired, nor should complimentary comments be made about its good looks or good health, lest some harm comes upon the child through the 'evil eye'.

RELIGIOUS BELIEFS AND PRACTICES

Bodily cleanliness is regarded in many cultures as a religious duty, and therefore in some sense a mark of piety. 'Cleanliness is next to godliness.' This obligation is expressed in personal cleanliness, not in environmental hygiene, as those who have shuddered in the public conveniences of other lands can testify. Hindus aim to bathe each morning in flowing water (not a stagnant bath!). They wash the anal region with water after defecation, and generally regard a menstruating woman as ritually unclean, so that in some traditions she may not even enter the kitchen to prepare food. The faeces or other bodily secretions of another person, particularly one of low caste, are considered highly 'unclean', polluting those who come in contact with them. Muslims, too, consider bodily cleanliness a virtue, and wash ritually before each of their daily prayer times. Muslim women take a ritual bath at the end of each menstrual period, after which they are able to resume intercourse. If asked the date of their last menstrual period these patients often give the date of the *last*, not the *first*, day.

These attitudes to cleanliness and pollution may make it very difficult for a patient to accept the idea of a bowel stoma, and faecal or urinary incontinence can create great distress, making the patient feel a virtual outcast. Because nurses have to deal with excreta, nursing may be seen as a degrading low-status occupation, and nurses may be accorded less respect for this reason.

Food and fasting play an important part in the religious life of many cultures. A Muslim will not partake of pork, and will eat other meat only if the animal was ritually slaughtered (*halal* meat). An orthodox Jew does not eat dairy products and meat at the same meal, and again his meat must be correctly slaughtered (*kosher*). Many Hindus are exclusively vegetarian and those who are not would generally not eat beef or pork. They may fast on particular holy days each week or month. During the lunar month of Ramadan, devout Muslims fast between sunrise and sunset. Although pregnant women are not obliged to fast during Ramadan, very many do so, from piety and a wish to share in the collective attestation of the observance.

These and other dietary observances can create great difficulty for the patient in hospital, who may refuse much of the food that is offered, and may prefer to eat only the food brought in by relatives. Apart from these more stringent observances, dietary choice may be restricted by other beliefs about food. In Indian culture it is generally held that some foods (vegetable oil, maize or millet flour, unrefined sugar, strong spices, onions) are 'hot', and therefore stimulating or even aphrodisiac, whereas others (milk, butter, wheat flour, rice, white sugar, honey) are 'cool', and so are safer and less disturbing. If sexual restraint (or even asceticism) is deemed a religious virtue and a prerequisite for good health, certain 'hot' foods may have to be avoided altogether.

In this context, it is important also to understand how loss of semen, whether from nocturnal emission, spermatorrhoea, masturbation or frequent coitus, has become in some Asian cultures a common source of sustained anxiety among males. In the ancient tradition of the Vedas, semen was considered to be a sort of vital essence, a source of psychic energy and well-being. It was said to be formed from blood, each drop of semen requiring forty drops of blood and forty days for its 'distillation'. As a legacy of these beliefs in some cultures, normal fatigue or impaired concentration may be construed as symptoms of depletion of semen, and anxious men may become obsessionally concerned about seminal loss. The complaint of passing a 'white substance' in the urine (*dhat* syndrome) is regularly encountered. The popularity of aphrodisiacs in various cultures also reflects underlying anxiety about loss of potency.

OTHER ATTITUDES TO FOOD

In many areas of the world most people are too poor to be able to afford a nourishing diet, and the really poor are evidently under-weight because of inadequate nutrition. Obesity is then naturally regarded as a cultural mark of affluence and social status, something to be proud of in one's self, one's spouse, and one's children. In this setting, advice to reduce weight is likely to be ignored.

There is reluctance in some cultures to give certain foods to young children. The banned foods often include eggs, milk, and fish, leading to protein deficiency.

In many folk traditions, dietary alterations are advocated for women during pregnancy. It is interesting that, while the recommended diets are likely to contain herbal and other supplements to help to ensure easy labour, it is unusual for a general calorie increase to be recommended. On the contrary, in several cultures (such as the tribes of the Arabian interior) the mother-to-be is deliberately deprived of high-calorie foods, with the professed aim of producing a less heavy infant, and a less difficult birth.

During breast-feeding, traditional food supplements are usually calorie-rich, and easily digestible. They may contain ginger, turmeric, and fenugreek.

ATTITUDES TO LIFE EVENTS: FATE AND DEATH

Most religions acknowledge the influence of a supernatural force or forces in the affairs of humankind. Devout believers, whether Christians, Muslims, or Hindus, feel their fate is in the hands of a higher being. Just as Christians may qualify their future plans with 'd.v.' (*Deo volente*), so Muslims, in speaking of future events, add '*ensh-Allah*' (if God wills), the same qualifying words. In Hindu culture, trust in astrology and horoscopes is strong, and auspicious dates may have to be chosen for surgical operations, or induction of labour. Behind this is belief in the recurring cycle of reincarnation, in the course of which the soul is inexorably requited or rewarded for behaviour in a previous life (*karma*). Those who are disabled may thus come to feel a sense of unworthiness, as if they had only received their just reward.

All these various influences tend to create an underlying feeling that a person's fate or destiny is pre-ordained, and that a wise man accepts his powerlessness to control or even influence events in his own life. Such fatalism can make easier the acceptance of suffering, death, bereavement, or disability—it provides a protective means of coping—but is also liable to engender a passivity towards events and to weaken any readiness to strive, overcome, or wrestle with the 'foul clutch of circumstance'.

The acceptance of death is not only a matter of fatalism. Death in the traditional cultures of some less developed countries is also accepted more readily because it is a common event in the past experience of the family, especially the death of children, and also because ready access to life-saving medical care is not the normal expectation.

The rituals of death and mourning among different religious faiths were well described by Black [54]. The head of a dying Muslim should be turned towards Mecca by moving the bed, and readings from the Koran performed. As soon as possible after death, the members of a Muslim family will wish to take the body, so that it can be ritually washed by the hands of believers, with prayers, and so prepared for burial, wrapped in a clean white sheet, on the same day if possible. Both Muslims and Hindus (but not Sikhs) hold that only fellow-believers should touch the dead body; others should wear gloves. After miscarriage, a Muslim couple will usually wish to treat the body of the fetus with similar respect, before burial.

Hindus often prefer to die at home, accompanied by prayers. The body is again washed ritually by family members, and so prepared for cremation. However, still births and children under the age of about four years are not usually cremated, but buried. The eldest son's participation in the funeral rites (whenever possible) is believed to be necessary for the true rest of the departed soul. After cremation, the ashes (in Britain) may be scattered over any large expanse of water. There is a prescribed period of 12 days mourning, during which white clothes are worn. Socially, grief and mourning are commonly expressed through rituals—vigils with the corpse, breast-beating, ululant wailing.

When death occurs, Muslims and orthodox Jews oppose post-mortem examination, and in other cultures too there is reluctance to allow the body of a dead relative to be mutilated in this way. For similar reasons, donation of organs, such as kidneys, may be quite unacceptable, except possibly for the benefit of a close relative. While the loyalties within the compound family are very strong, they can also be somewhat insular. As a result, the sense of social obligation to give blood (for example) may be limited to the family, or the clan or caste group. Besides, among some traditional Muslims the transfusion of blood may be thought to bring about a permanent new 'blood' relationship between the donor and the recipient. Breast-feeding has a similar significance, and so the giving or receiving of breast-milk through a bank may be unacceptable.

HEALTH BELIEFS AND PRACTICES

Every community has a varied store of traditional homely remedies, especially for common ailments. In many cultures, a more formal system of traditional medicine exists, with its own explanations of how the body functions, and what promotes health or causes illness. The practitioners may have acquired their knowledge and skills through apprenticeship or by more systematic instruction. The ancient systems of Chinese and Indian (Ayurvedic) medicine rely heavily on herbal preparations, but also utilize exotic remedies prepared from animal products, precious stones, or metals, for example. African traditional medicine encompasses a wide range of practitioners, including bone-setters, surgeons, and manipulators, as well as spirit-healers. Exorcism has been seen as an occasional remedy in Britain and other countries for many centuries past.

In Chinese traditional therapeutics, acupuncture plays an important part. Just as Roman Catholics might wear St. Christopher medallions, and fundamentalist Protestants have their promise boxes packed with reassuring Biblical verses, in Islamic communities amulets containing verses from the Koran are commonly worn as a protection from illness, and traditional therapy may include a potion prepared by washing a Koranic verse from a slate. Moxibustion, cupping, blood-letting (*hijaam*), and cauterization (*wassum*), are other older methods of traditional therapy.

Much nearer home, what are generally known as 'alternative therapies' (see the BMA report [114]) have become fashionable in recent years. These include osteopathy, chiropractic, homoeopathy, herbalism, massage, aromatherapy, reflexology, yoga, and faith healing. Even in a culture in which scientific medicine holds strong sway over people's minds and outlooks, some individuals seek health or healing through different modalities of treatment, in certain cases based on quite bizarre beliefs.

In health terms, some social practices of other cultures are rightly censured as harmful and mutilative, for example female circumcision; *geshiri* vaginal cutting (Northern Nigeria). To maintain perspective it is necessary also to recognize the harmful social compulsions existing in our own culture, ranging from skin damage induced by tanning to liposculpture and eating disorders.

Sometimes patients from a traditional culture may feel it wise to aim for the best of both worlds, and so consult an orthodox practitioner while concurrently seeking the advice of a traditional healer, or taking a traditional remedy on their own initiative. Often their ability to assimilate information and to follow medical instructions depends on their being able to translate the information into a form which fits in with their traditional health beliefs, and their understanding of how the body works. Some patients from other cultures who adopt Western medicine show reluctance to place full trust in the opinion of a single doctor. They may consult independently two or three doctors, or even more if they have the means, as if the best advice would emerge from a sort of ballot of medical opinion. Their behaviour, if brought into the open, is likely to antagonize the doctors concerned, because of the implied lack of confidence.

What appears to be distrust of doctors can sometimes be shown by American patients, because of the manner in which they are liable to interrogate the doctor over seeming minutiae, may expect multiple laboratory tests to validate the diagnosis, and demand something more than the usual explanation for each step in management. Often this appearance of distrust is little more than a desire for greater and more informed involvement in matters concerning the individual's health, but it may be intensified because the patient's attitude has been influenced by the commercialism of some American practice.

In contrast, many patients from developing countries (whether because of limited education, misplaced respectfulness, or just acquiescence) are likely to ask no questions of the doctor, and seek no explanation of his advice. Doctors trained in this sort of setting often have little skill in exposition, and limited awareness of the importance of patient education, explanation, and other facets of good communication.

This short chapter provides no more than a few illustrative glimpses of various cultural patterns and practices, and of the way in which these can affect communication between patient and doctor. The student who aims to communicate better, and to understand more about patients' feelings, attitudes, and behaviour, needs to broaden his knowledge of cultures other than his own. Empathy, on which good communication so vitally depends, rests on the doctor's awareness of what is going on in the patient's mind. This presents a much more difficult challenge when cultural boundaries have to be crossed.

21 Developing the skills

A central theme of this book is the message that skill in interviewing is essentially a product of professional learning, rather than an innate ability that some possess from birth, but others lack. It is sometimes claimed that students should be selected for admission to medical schools partly on the basis of their ability to communicate, that only 'outgoing' personalities should be accepted, in the hope that all doctors would, almost automatically, turn out to be good communicators. Perhaps some form of personality and aptitude testing might be a fruitful part of the selection process, rather than reliance solely on the student's ability to score well in a narrow range of science subjects in school qualifying exams. However, given the range of careers a medical graduate may pursue—in clinical, administrative, laboratory, investigative, or military medicine, for example—it would be difficult to specify the particular qualities to be required in every entrant. In all these fields communication skills are of great value, even though the doctors concerned may not be in day-to-day contact with patients.

UNFAVOURABLE INFLUENCES

There is evidence that the process of undergraduate medical education may, in some instances, inhibit rather than promote the development of interviewing skills. One or two studies have shown this effect [115,116], which might be a consequence of the traditional pre-clinical/clinical divide in the medical curriculum. If a student is 'imprinted' with a conceptual framework of function and disease based solely on the physical sciences, he may acquire a view of patients as disordered machines before he even begins to learn to talk to them as people, particularly if his main early contacts with the subject of study have been as a cadaver in the dissecting room, or at autopsy.

There is no doubt that early and continuing contact with patients is important in promoting the facility for good communication. At this stage, there is little correlation between students' confidence in themselves and their actual ability to communicate well; females tend to do better than males [117]. But when the student does start regular clinical work in the wards, he may be presented with a poor model of doctor–patient communication during traditional ward rounds. As the hierarchical retinue of doctors, students, and nurses processes around the ward, communication with patients may well be overshadowed by the intra-professional exchanges at the foot of the bed, where the medical staff are, it has to be admitted, often preoccupied with a professionally centred game of

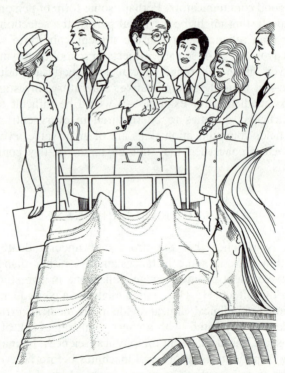

Fig 21.1 The ward round: a frequent example of poor communication

one-up-manship, which Arluke has called 'roundsmanship' [118] (Fig. 21.1). Viewed cynically, the motives evident may be to impress, flatter, or deceive the 'chief'; to score off the sister or the registrar; or to demonstrate and reinforce the pecking order to the students!

Some pitfalls and obstacles that can stand in the way of good communication during ward rounds have been well described by Steele and Morton [119]. They include lack of privacy, inadequate explanation, and open criticism of staff or students, as well as behaviour such as ignoring or excluding the patient, and 'exhibiting' the patient. Not uncommonly the intra-professional exchanges in the course of a ward round are couched in language which is ultratechnical, or deliberately obscure so that the patient cannot readily eavesdrop:

'The chest film shows pulmonary neoplasia with extensive metastases.'
'We're definitely thinking this may be a supratentorial problem.'
'Our concern about the hyperkalaemia is that unheralded ventricular asystole may occur.'

From language of this sort, the student may acquire more skill in concealing or fudging than in communicating.

ACTIVE DEVELOPMENT OF INTERVIEWING SKILLS

Students can best develop their skill in interviewing by participating in or observing, and then discussing, actual interviews. This learning process is most fruitful when conducted in a small group of (say) six to eight students with a tutor. If resources allow, two students with a tutor can refine specific skills. The opportunities for detailed learning are greatly enhanced if the interviews can be recorded on videotape (or even audiotape) so that, with playback, precise recall and review of the exchanges during each interview are possible. Video methods, of course, also allow the non-verbal elements in the interaction between doctor and patient to be studied carefully [120] and are therefore much more valuable than the use of audiotapes alone.

Initially, students may feel self-conscious at the prospect of their awkwardness being laid bare in front of their fellow students. The tutor needs to arrange that all members of the group are equally 'exposed'; that unfair criticisms are countered; and that positive feedback and encouragement is the order of the day.

Aims and guidelines for the group therefore need to be clearly set out. Only within a secure, confidential, and mutually trusting environment are students likely to express their ignorance, anxiety, and other concerns. As they begin to recognize that each of them has something to offer within the circle of the group, and that what they say will be taken seriously by the leader, even the habitually silent 'listeners' will be encouraged to contribute, and their self-esteem will be enhanced [121,122].

When this format of learning is being used, one of the students takes the part of the doctor, while the 'patient' may be a real patient who has consented to participate. Many patients are happy to assist in this way if the purpose of the exercise is carefully explained to them, because of their awareness of the importance of improving doctors' communication skills. Alternatively, a simulated patient can be used. This individual may be a medical teacher or a lay volunteer (possibly an amateur actor) who has been briefed to play a particular patient role. If the volunteer remains 'in role' during the subsequent discussion, he can provide direct feed back to students about how their approach felt to the 'patient'. But he needs to do this in a sensitive, encouraging way.

However, excellent opportunities for new learning during this type of exercise can occur when a second student plays the role of the patient, or relative, guided by a brief written in advance. The student entering into the role of a patient has to reflect on how that patient would feel and behave in a particular situation, and so his capacity for empathy develops and his learning can be shared with other students in the group [123].

Other advantages of using a simulated patient are that the real patients are not inconvenienced and the tutor can freely choose the clinical problem on which the group will centre, rather than being confined to the range of clinical cases present within the ward or clinic on that particular day.

FURTHER LEARNING

We have reviewed the skills of affective communication in the general context of everyday consultations with a variety of patients.

There are additional skills that need to be used in specific situations, for instance with blind patients, deaf or aphasic patients, or those who can be spoken to only through an interpreter. In other sections of the book, the problems of affective communication that arise in caring for dying patients, or in helping the patient with sexual difficulties, have been described. Again, specific skills are called for in these situations. There is always more to learn!

I have deliberately not sought to explore in detail those dimensions of dialogue that are generally referred to as 'counselling', in which an important aim is to assist the client/patient to resolve for himself difficulties in his relationships with others, to make well-informed decisions about his life, and in the process to reach a greater degree of self-understanding and self-reliance. Similarly, I have not called upon the interpretive constructs of the doctor–patient relationship derived from depth psychology (psycho-analysis), as expounded by Balint and his school [124]. In pursuing these approaches, the doctor should undertake a period of further training, submitting his own attitudes and feelings to open self and peer-group scrutiny.

Not all doctors have the time, inclination, or aptitude to adopt these models of patient–doctor interaction. I have attempted to outline a less sophisticated approach, appropriate for everyday practice, using concepts and frames of reference with which the student is likely to be familiar. Certain inhibitory influences that must be recognized and overcome, especially by students learning interviewing skills at the basic level, are identified. It is my hope that an understanding of these factors will promote improved interviewing skills and the adoption of a more sensitive and empathic clinical style. In consequence, tomorrow's medical graduates may be less likely to evoke from their patients the sorts of justifiable criticism that were discussed at the outset. At the same time, they will enhance their clinical problem-solving skills in line with the need so clearly spelt out in the report 'Physicians for the Twentyfirst Century' [125], and reiterated in the King's Fund study (1991) 'Critical thinking: the future of undergraduate medical education.'

Résumé

The purpose of this book has been to demonstrate that effective sensitive communication calls for specific skills, which can be defined through analysis of actual interviews and developed through understanding and practice. It is a fallacy to rely on just being one's self—on being 'natural'. In fact, the spontaneous human feelings that are liable to be evoked during dialogue with patients, whether feelings of sympathy or aversion, attraction or repulsion, have to be controlled and modified by the doctor's professionalism.

When these professional skills are well deployed, the effect is not to isolate the doctor from the patient. On the contrary, a clinical setting is created within which the doctor feels secure enough to reduce the distance between himself and the patient while retaining an appropriate and necessary degree of professional detachment. At the same time, the patient is helped to voice feelings and concerns that might otherwise have remained unexpressed [126].

Detachment and involvement are both, in a measure, necessary attributes of the professional's role. But it is fair to say that, in seeking a balance between them, doctors have inclined traditionally towards detachment. Maintaining a greater distance from the patient can appear very attractive. It reinforces the doctor's authority; it insulates a doctor from the patient's pain or other distress; it helps to dissociate the doctor from any possible sense of failure. Involvement, in contrast, can seem rather threatening and burdensome. It might put pressure on the doctor beyond his capacity; it might create discomfort in coping with emotions; it could eventually culminate in 'burn-out' if the doctor allowed his involvement to become too intense or too prolonged.

I have endeavoured in this volume to outline a professional attitude and manner that avoids either extreme, and which therefore has, I believe, a better claim to the epithet 'professional'. It aims to meet the expectation voiced by many patients at the present time that their doctors should not just be competent diagnosticians and good technicians (however important that may be) but should also bring to their work the skills and attitudes of caring. This implies, above all, the sort of sensitive and open interpersonal communication that I and my contributors have sought to describe.

Appendix

SYSTEMATIC OUTLINE OF TOPICS WHICH MAY NEED TO BE REVIEWED IN A COMPREHENSIVE MEDICAL HISTORY

This outline is based on guidance notes given to medical students at the University of Edinburgh, under the auspices of the Medical Education Committee.

First, list the patient's *presenting complaints*, as far as possible in his own words. Give a brief chronological narrative of their onset. It may be necessary to interview a third party in the case of children; confused, inebriated, or unconscious patients; and those suffering from severe emotional disorders or mental illness.

The *characteristics of each symptom* should be defined in some detail.

- duration;
- mode of onset—sudden or gradual;
- possible association, e.g. exercise, meals, movement, emotional tension;
- periodicity—nocturnal pattern, interference with sleep;
- progression;
- localization;
- premonitory, precipitating, aggravating, or relieving factors;
- effect on patient's everyday life: patient's reaction to the complaint.

Past medical history

Previous illnesses, operations and other health problems should be listed, with a note of the date or patient's age at the time. Remember that inaccuracies and omissions are common.

Note prominently any hypersensitivity to drugs, X-ray contrast media, or other agents.

Drug history

Identify all current medication, and all treatment previously given for the present illness. Was it effective? Were there any abnormal reactions?

Alcohol consumption should be estimated quantitatively. What is the pattern of drinking? Is there evidence of dependence?

Smoking: present and past habits. Is there any other 'social' drug use?

Obstetric history (females)

State the total number of pregnancies and abortions. Note complications of pregnancy or labour. Enquire about the current health of any children. Note the method(s) of contraception used, if any.

Comprehensive enquiry: checklist of more common symptoms

Symptoms not present can be recorded thus: dyspnoea—0.

General

Weight loss or gain, energy, sleep pattern, general well-being—if vague, enquire 'When did you last feel well?'

Cardiovascular system
- Dyspnoea
- Ankle oedema
- Chest pain—on exertion or at rest
- Palpitations
- Intermittent claudication

Respiratory system
- Cough; sputum (colour, amount)
- Dyspnoea; wheeze
- Haemoptysis
- Chest pain

Gastrointestinal system

- Appetite; dietary pattern
- Weight change
- Dysphagia
- Indigestion; heartburn; waterbrash
- Postprandial pain
- Nausea; vomiting
- Abdominal pain—continuous/colicky
- Bowel habit—constipation/diarrhoea; recent change; stools—blood/pallor/odour/mucus/incontinence
- Jaundice

Renal and genitourinary system

- Thirst
- Micturition—frequency; polyuria; nocturia
- Dysuria; hesitancy; impaired stream; urgency
- Incontinence—stress/urge/complete
- Haematuria; urine colour/frothiness
- Lumbar or loin pain
- Balanitis; urethral discharge
- Sexual function
  in men—impotence; premature ejaculation
  in women—dyspareunia; impaired desire or response
- (Women) Menstrual function
  age of menarche; cycle length; duration and amount of menstrual flow
  date of last period
  if no longer menstruating, date of menopause; any menopausal symptoms; any post-menopausal bleeding
  leukorrhoea; pruritus vulvae

Central nervous system

- Impaired vision—acuity/field of vision/diplopia
- Impaired hearing; tinnitus
- Fainting/fits/black-outs/dizziness/vertigo
- Headaches; loss of consciousness
- Loss of sensation; paraesthesiae
- Paralysis; paresis
- Mood impairment; sleep pattern; early-morning waking

Skin

- Itching (pruritus)
- Rashes; eruptions—petechiae—bruising
- Contact with plants, pets, etc.
- Occupational/recreational skin irritants

Locomotor system

- Impaired mobility
- Difficulty in walking—limp/unsteadiness/loss of balance
- Backache
- Joint pain or swelling
- Muscle pain—cramps—weakness
- Postures or activities that relieve or aggravate the pain
- Use of sticks or other aids

FAMILY HISTORY

Review all first-degree relatives (parents, children, siblings). Record present age and state of health. If dead, state cause, and reactions to bereavement in the family. Note occurrence of similar or associated disease within the family.

Social history

This should encompass the following.

- the patient's household circumstances and occupational environment;
- some impression of the patient's lifestyle;
- interpersonal relationships at home and at work;
- occupational history—employed/unemployed; stability of job tenure; occupational hazards;
- travel abroad—alone/with partner; countries visited. In some instances, sexual contacts abroad will be relevant.
- pets, flocks, herds—other close contacts with animals or birds.

References

1. Nuffield Provincial Hospitals Trust (1980). *Talking with patients: a teaching approach*. Oxford University Press.
2. Stiles, W.B. *et al.* (1979). Interaction exchange structure and patient satisfaction with medical interviews. *Medical Care*, **17**, 667–81.
3. Comstock, L.M. *et al.* (1982). Physician behaviours that correlate with patient satisfaction. *Journal of Medical Education*, **57**, 105–12.
4. Korsch, B.M., Gozzi, E.K., and Francis, V. (1968). Doctor–patient interaction and patient satisfaction. *Paediatrics*, **42**, 855–71.
5. Sandler, G. (1979). Costs of unnecessary tests. *British Medical Journal*, **2**, 21–4.
6. Hampton, J.R. *et al.* (1975). Relative contribution of history-taking, physical examination and laboratory investigations to diagnosis and management of medical outpatients. *British Medical Journal*, **2**, 486–9.
7. Fletcher, C. (1980). Listening and talking to patients, III. The exposition. *British Medical Journal*, **2**, 994–6.
8. Enelow, A.J. and Swisher, S.N. (1986). *Interviewing and patient care*, (3rd edn). Oxford University Press.
9. Cartwright, A. (1964). *Human relations and hospital care*. Routledge & Kegan Paul, London.
10. Dunkelmans, H. (1979). Patients' knowledge of their condition and treatment: how it might be improved. *British Medical Journal*, **2**, 311.
11. Hawkins, C. (1979). Patient's reactions to their investigations. *British Medical Journal* **2**, 638–40.
12. Parkin, D.M. (1976). Survey of the success of communication between hospital staff and patients. *Public Health*, **90**, 203–9.
13. Reynolds, M. (1978). No news is bad news: patients' views about communication in hospital. *British Medical Journal*, **1**, 1673.
14. Ley, P. (1983). In *Doctor–patient communication*, (ed. D. Pendleton and J. Hasler), pp. 89–107. Academic Press, London.
15. Report of the Health Service Commissioner for 1991–2. (1993). HMSO, London.
16. McNamara, M. (1974). Talking with patients: some problems met by medical students. *British Journal of Medical Education*, **8**, 17–23.
17. Firth-Cozens, J. (1987). Emotional distress in junior house-officers. *British Medical Journal*, **295**, 533–36.
18. Flexner, A. (1910). *Medical education in the U.S.A. and Canada. A*

report for the Carnegie Foundation for the Advancement of Teaching, Bull. No. 4. Updike, Boston, MA; reprinted (1972) Arno Press.

19. Pendleton, D., Schofield, T., Tate, T., and Havelock, P. (1990). *The consultation: an approach to learning and teaching.* Oxford University Press.

20. Asher, R. (1972). *Richard Asher talking sense*, p. 170. Pitman Medical, London.

21. Meadows, R. (1977). Munchausen syndrome by proxy: the hinterland of child abuse. *Lancet*, **2**, 343–5.

22. Maguire, P. (1985). Barriers to the psychological care of the dying. *British Medical Journal*, **291**, 1711.

23. Wilson-Barnett, J. (1989). In *Psychological management of the physically ill*, (ed. J.H. Lacey and T. Burns). Churchill-Livingstone, Edinburgh.

24. Morris, D. (1978). *Manwatching. A field guide to human behaviour.* Panther Books, London.

25. Maguire, G.P. and Rutter, D.R. (1976). In *Communication between doctors and patients*, (ed. A.E. Bennett). Oxford University Press.

26. Billings, J.A. and Stoekle, J.D. (1989). *The clinical encounter: a guide to the medical interview and case presentation.* Year Book, Chicago, IL.

27. Macartney, F.J. (1987). Diagnostic logic. *British Medical Journal*, **295**, 1325–33.

28. Kassirer, J.P. (1989). Our stubborn quest for diagnostic certainty: a cause of excessive testing. *New England Journal of Medicine*, **320**, 1489–91.

29. Barrows, H.S. (1973). *Problem-based learning in medicine*, Educational Monograph No. 4. McMaster University, Hamilton, Ontario.

30. Elstein, A.S. *et al.* (1978). *Medical problem-solving: an analysis of clinical reasoning.* Harvard University Press, Cambridge, MA.

31. Barrows, H.S. *et al.* (1978). *An analysis of the clinical methods of medical students and physicians.* McMaster University, Hamilton, Ontario.

32. Campbell, E.J.M. (1976). Basic science, science and medical education. *Lancet*, **1**, 134–6.

33. Campbell, E.J.M. (1976). Clinical science and medical education. *Clinical Science and Molecular Medicine*, **51**, 1–7.

34. De Dombal, F.T. *et al.* (1972). Computer-aided diagnosis of acute abdominal pain. *British Medical Journal*, **2**, 9–13.

35. De Dombal, F.T. *et al.* (1974). Human and computer-aided diagnosis of abdominal pain. *British Medical Journal*, **2**, 376–80.

36. Warner, H.R., Toronto, A.F., Veasy, L.G., and Stephenson, R.S. (1961). A mathematical approach to medical diagnosis: application to

congenital heart disease. *Journal of the American Medical Association*, **177**, 177–83.
37. (a) Edelwich, J. and Brodsky, A. (1980). *Burn-out: stages of disillusionment in the helping professions*. Human Sciences Press, New York. (b) Roberts, G.A. (1986). Burn-out; psycho-babble or valuable concept? *British Journal of Hospital Medicine*, **36**, 194.
38. Buchanan, J.H. (1989). *Patient encounters: the experience of disease*. University Press of Virginia, Charlottesville, VI.
39. Patients Association (1982). *Self help and the patient*. A directory of national organisations concerned with particular diseases and handicaps. Patients Association. London.
40. (a) Todd, J. *et al.* (1982). *Someone to talk to; a directory of self-help groups and support services in the community*. Thames TV in association with the Mental Health Foundation, London. (b) The *Coping with* series (1985). Chambers, London. (c) The *Overcoming common problems* series. (1985). Sheldon Press, London.
41. Morell, D.C. *et al.* (1986). The 'five-minute' consultation: effect of time-constraint on clinical content and patient satisfaction. *British Medical Journal*, **292**, 870–73.
42. Roland, M.O. *et al.* (1986). The 'five-minute' consultation: effect of time constraint on verbal communication. *British Medical Journal*, **292**, 874–6.
43. Eimeri, T.S. and Pearson, R.J.C. (1966). Working time in general practice: how general practitioners use their time. *British Medical Journal*, **2**, 1549–54.
44. Stott, N.C.H. and Davis, R.H. (1979). The exceptional potential in each primary care consultation. *Journal of the Royal College of General Practitioners*, **29**, 201–5.
45. Wilkinson, C. (1989). Uninterrupted speaking of patient in general practice and consultant clinic. *British Medical Journal*, **298**, 389.
46. Seravalli, P. (1988). The dying patient, the physician, and the fear of death. *New England Journal of Medicine*, **319**, 1728–30.
47. Maguire, P. (1989). In *Psychological management of the physically ill*, (ed. J.H. Lacey and T. Burns), pp. 193–212. Churchill-Livingstone, Edinburgh.
48. Charlton, R. (1994). Personal view: Words of sorrow. *Student British Medical Journal* **2**, 42.
49. Hinton, J.M. (1972). *Dying*, (2nd edn). Penguin Books, London. [See also *British Medical Journal* (1980), **281**, 1328]
50. Kubler-Ross, E. (1970). *On death and dying*. Macmillan, New York.
51. Lewis, E. (1976). The management of stillbirth—coping with an unreality. *Lancet*, **2**, 619.
52. Bourne, S. (1968). The psychological effects of stillbirths on women

and their doctors. *Journal of the Royal College of General Practitioners*, **16**, 103.

53. Marley, J. (1989). Grief and how to manage it. *Practitioner*, **233**, 287–9.
54. Black, J. (1987). Broaden your mind about death and bereavement in certain ethnic groups in Britain. *British Medical Journal*, **295**, 536–9.
55. Health Education Council (1981). *The loss of your baby*. [In co-operation with the National Association for Mental Health and the National Stillbirth Study Group]
56. Leroy, M. (1988). *Miscarriage*. Macdonald Optima, London.
57. Friedman, T. (1989). Women's experience of general practitioners' management of miscarriage. *Journal of the Royal College of General Practitioners*, **39**, 456–8.
58. Cook, B. and Phillips, S.G. (1988) *Loss and Bereavement*. Austen Cornish. London.
59. Black, D., Hardoff, D., and Nelki, J. (1989). Educating medical students about death and dying. *Archives of the Diseases of Childhood*, **64**, 750–3.
60. Fahy, T. and Fisher, N. (1992). Sexual contact between doctors and patients. *British Medical Journal*, **304**, 1519; 1531–4.
61. Jones, R. (1993). Use of chaperones. *British Medical Journal*, **307**, 951–2.
62. Jones, R.H. (1983). The use of chaperones by general practitioners. *Journal of the Royal College of General Practitioners*, **33**, 25.
63. Van Beukesom, J.A.H. (1973). In *Anxiety factors in comprehensive patient care*, (ed. W.L. Rees), pp. 26–31. Excerpta Medica, Amsterdam.
64. Jeffrey, D. (1993). *'There is nothing more I can do': an introduction to the ethics of palliative care*. Patten Press, Penzance.
65. Buckman, R. (1984). Breaking bad news. *British Medical Journal*, **288**, 597.
66. Brewin, T.B. (1991). Three ways of giving bad news. *Lancet*, **337**, 1207–9.
67. Hogbin, B. and Fallowfield, L. (1989). Getting it taped; the bad news consultation with cancer patients. *British Journal of Hospital Medicine*, **41**, 330–3.
68. Thrush, D.C. (1993). Epilepsy: clinical management. *Proceeding of the Royal College of Physicians, Edinburgh*, **23**, 455–62.
69. Hughes, R.A.C. (1993). The management of multiple sclerosis. *Proceedings of the Royal College of Physicians*, Edinburgh, **23**, 446–54.
70. Weatherall, D.J. (1994). The inhumanity of medicine. *British Medical Journal*, **309**, 1671–2.
71. Guidance on patient consent (1990). H.C. (90) 22. HMSO, London.

72. *The Patients Charter*. Department of Health (1991). HMSO, London.
73. Lewis, P.J.D., O'Keefe, L., and Adcock, S. (1991), (letter). *Journal of the Royal College of Surgeons, Edinburgh*, **36**, 206–7.
74. Ward, M. (1990). Letter from Australia: ways of looking at the world. *Proceedings of the Royal College of Physicians of Edinburgh*, **20**, 64–6.
75. Slevin, M.L. *et al.* (1990). Attitudes to chemotherapy; comparing views of patients with cancer to those of doctors and nurses and the general public. *British Medical Journal*, **300**, 1458–60.
76. Dear, P.R.F. (1989). Attitudes to the risk of adverse neonatal outcome. *Contemporary Reviews in Obstetrics and Gynaecology*, **1**, 207–13.
77. Ley, P. (1982). Satisfaction, compliance and communication. *British Journal of Clinical Psychology*, **21**, 241–54.
78. Korsch, B.M. and Negretti, V.F. (1972). Doctor–patient communication. *Scientific American*, **227** (No. 2), 66–71.
79. Bradley, C. (1993). Quoted in *The Independent*, p. 20. 14 September.
80. Sandler, D.A., Mitchell, J.R.A., Fellows, A., and Garner, S.T. (1989). Is an information booklet for patients leaving hospital helpful and useful? *British Medical Journal*, **293**, 870–4.
81. Sandler, D.A., Heaton, C., Garner, S.T., and Mitchell, J.R.A. (1989). Patients' and general practitioners' satisfaction with information given on discharge from hospital: audit of a new information card. *British Medical Journal*, **299**, 1511–13.
82. Cornblett, M.A. *et al.* (1992) Recording of out patient consultations (letter). *Lancet*, **340**, 488.
83. Read, G. (1992), Consultants communications with G.P.s. *British Medical Journal*, **304**, 1248.
84. Ridout, S., Waters, W.E., and George, C.F. (1986). Knowledge of and attitudes to medicines in the Southhampton community. *British Journal of Clinical Pharmacology*, **21**, 701–12.
85. Anand, K.J.S. (1985). Can the human neonate mount an endocrine and metabolic response to surgery? *Journal of Paediatric Surgery*, **20**, 41–80.
86. Anand, K.J.S. (1987). Randomised trial of fentanyl anaesthesia in preterm babies undergoing surgery: effects on the stress response. *Lancet*, (1987), **1**, 62–6
87. Anand, K.J.S. (1992). Halothane–morphine compared with high dose sufentanil for anaesthesia and postoperative analgesia in neonatal cardiac surgery. *New England Journal of Medicine*, **326**, 397–405.
88. Field, T. *et al.* (1986). Tactile/kinesthetic stimulation on preterm neonates. *Pediatrics*, **77**, 654–8.

89. Boston, S. (1981). *Will, my son. The life and death of a mongol child.* Pluto Press, London.
90. Laing, I.A. (1989). Withdrawing from invasive neonatal intensive care. In *Paediatric forensic medicine and pathology*, (ed. J.K. Mason). Chapman & Hall, London.
91. *Report of the Inquiry into Child Abuse in Cleveland*, 1987 (1988). HMSO, London.
92. Murray, K. and Gough, D.A. (1991). *Intervening in child sexual abuse.* Scottish Academic Press, Edinburgh.
93. Wooley, H., Stern, A., Forrest, G.C., and Baum, J.D. (1989). Imparting the diagnosis of life threatening illness in children. *British Medical Journal*, **298**, 1623–6.
94. Blos, P. (1967). The second individuation phase of adolescence. In *Psychoanalytic study of the child*, Vol. 22. International University Press, New York.
95. Evans, J. (1982). *Adolescent and pre-adolescent psychiatry.* Academic Press, London.
96. Coleman, J.C. (1980). *The nature of adolescence.* Methuen, London.
97. Offer, D. and Offer, J. (1975). Three developmental routes through adolescence. In *Adolescent psychiatry*, Vol. IV (ed. S.C. Feinstein and P.L. Giovacchini). Jason Aronson, New York.
98. Green, R. (1985). Atypical psycho-sexual development. *Child and adolescent psychiatry: modern approach*, (2nd edn) (ed. M. Rutter and L. Hersov). Blackwell Scientific, Oxford.
99. Erikson, E.H. (1950). *Childhood and society.* Norton, New York.
100. Rutter, M., Maughan, B., Mortimore, P., Ounston, J., and Smith, A. (1979). *Fifteen thousand hours: Secondary schools and their effect on children.* Open Books, London.
101. Weatherley, D. (1964). Self-perceived rate of physical maturation and personality in late adolescence. *Child Development*, **35**, 1107–210.
102. Will, D. and Wrate, R.M. (1985). *Integrated family therapy: a problem-centred psychodynamic approach.* Tavistock Publications, London.
103. Cox, A., Holbrook, D., and Rutter, M. (1981). Psychiatric interviewing techniques. VI. Experimental study: eliciting feelings. *British Journal of Psychiatry*, **139**, 144–52.
104. Hawton, K., Osborn, M., O'Grady, J., and Cole, D. (1982). Adolescents who take overdoses: their characteristics, problems and contacts with helping agencies. *British Journal of Psychiatry*, **140**, 118–23.
105. Mrazek, P.B. and Bentovim, A. (1981). Incest and the dysfunctional family system. In *Sexually abused children and their families* (ed. P.B. Mrazek and C.H. Kempe). Pergamon Press, London.
106. Morrison, J., Roberts, J., and Will, D. (1987). Twenty myths that

justify not investigating child sexual abuse. *Social Work Today*, July 20.

107. Jaemmet, A. (1981). The anorexic stance. *Journal of Adolescence*, **4**, 113–19.

108. Minuchin, S. (1974). *Families and family therapy*. Tavistock Publications, London.

109. Bastian, H. (1992). Confined, managed and delivered: the language of obstetrics. *British Journal of Obstetrics and Gynaecology*, **99**, 92–3.

110. Davies, V. (1991). *Abortion and afterwards*. Ashgrove Press. Bath.

111. Hawkes, C.H. (1974). Communicating with the patient—an example drawn from neurology. *British Journal of Medical Education*, **8**, 57–63.

112. Littlewood, R. and Lipsedge, M. (1985). Culture-bound syndromes. In *Recent advances in clinical psychiatry*, (ed. K. Granville-Grossman), p. 105. Churchill Livingstone, Edinburgh.

113. Rosenfield, M. and Maine, D. (1985). Maternal mortality: a neglected tragedy. *Lancet*, **2**, 83.

114. British Medical Association (1986). Report of the Board of Science working party on alternative therapy. *British Medical Journal*, **292**, 1407.

115. Poole, A.D. and Sanson-Fisher, R.W. (1979). Understanding the patient: a neglected aspect of medical education. *Social Sciences and Medicine*, **13A**, 37–43.

116. Helfer, R.E. and Ealy, K.F. (1972). Observation of paediatric interviewing skills. *American Journal of Diseases in Children*, **123**, 556–60.

117. Marteau, T.M. *et al.* (1991). Factors influencing the communication skills of first year clinical medical students. *Medical Education*, **25**, 127–34.

118. Arluke, E. (1980). Roundsmanship: inherent control on a medical teaching round. *Social Sciences and Medicine*, **14**, 297–302.

119. Steele, S.J. and Morton, D.J.B. (1978). The ward round. *Lancet*, **2**, 85–6.

120. Afsal Mir, M. *et al.* (1986). Video and audio-tapes for teaching history-taking. *Medical Education*, **20**, 102–8.

121. McManus, I.C. *et al.* (1993). Teaching communication skills to clinical students. *British Medical Journal*, **306**, 1322–27.

122. McAvoy, B.R. (1988) Teaching clinical skills to medical students: the use of simulated patients and videotaping in general practice. *Medical Education*, **22**, 193–6.

123. Van Ments, M. (1983). *The effective use of role-play. A handbook for teachers and trainers*. Kogan Page, London.

124. Balint, M. (1957). *The doctor, his patient and the illness*. Pitman, London.
125. *Physicians for the twentyfirst century*. The GPEP Report (1984). Association of American Medical Colleges, Washington, D.C.
126. Millar, T. and Goldberg, D.P. (1991). Link between the ability to detect and to manage emotional disorders: a study of general practitioner trainees. *British Journal of General Practice*, **41**, 357–9.
127. Goodwin, J. (1995). The importance of clinical skills. *British Medical Journal*, **310**, 1281–2.
128. *The psychological care of medical patients: Recognition of need and service provision*. Report (1995). Royal College of Physicians, London.
129. Schön, D.A. (1987). *Educating the reflective practitioner*. Jossey Bass Higher Educational Series, San Francisco and London.
130. Zigmond, A. and Snaith, R.P. (1983). The Hospital Anxiety and Depression Scale. *Acta Psychiatrica Scandinavica*, **67**, 361–70.

Index